LIFE-MASTERING HABIT TRACKER

TASHAI LOVINGTON

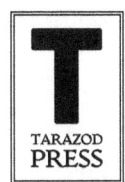

TARAZOD
PRESS

For more by Tashai Lovington, go to her website at: https://tashai.net

Cover design: © 2023 by Tashai J Lovington

Copyright 2023 by Tarazod Press LLC

ISBN: 979-8-9861947-2-1 (softcover)

PRAISE FOR TASHAI LOVINGTON

"I think a lot of people need to take advantage of this. I'm thrilled that you are doing the work, because it's so needed."
- **Jack Canfield**, New York Times Best Selling Author of The Success Principles and Co-creator of the #1 Best Selling book series Chicken Soup for the Soul

"This book is the secret weapon and blueprint that every person or professional can use to achieve happiness and success in their business, their career and in their life. Tashai Lovington has put together a unique collection of life's lessons, and success strategies to help you be the best person you can be. Her book is incredibly noteworthy, valuable and inspiring to help you learn how to never give up on yourself, overcome challenges and shine your life to the fullest now! "Fill The Gap" is truly magical! Well done!"
—**John Formica,** The "Ex-Disney Guy", America's customer experience speaker at JohnFormica.com

"This wonderful book shows you how to unlock your full potential and get the very most out of yourself." —**Brian Tracy**, President of Brian Tracy International and author "Maximum Achievement" and "Eat That Frog"

"These concepts are fundamental for those looking to get the life they've always dreamed of."
—**Kevin Harrington**, Original Shark from Shark Tank

"Tashai teaches you to believe in yourself and that the universe has your back." - **Patty Aubery**, #1 New York Times Best-selling author, Chicken Soup for the Christian Soul

"Tashai is so encouraging and inspires you to live a better life!" —**James Malinchak,** featured on ABC's Hit TV show, "Secret Millionaire", Founder, www.BigMoneySpeaker.com

"Take your life to the next level! Tashai offers invaluable techniques and exercises to !nally achieve the success you've always wanted" —**Jill Lublin**, Master Publicity, Strategist, 4x best-selling author.

"Tashai has laid the foundation for you with her tips, ideas and strategies. Her book should empower you to strive for greatness." —**Joe Theismann**, World Champion and Entrepreneur

MOTIVATE AND INSPIRE OTHERS!

"Share this Book"

Special quantity discounts

5-20 books $15.99
21-99 books $13.99
100-499 books $11.99
500-999 books $9.99
1000+ books $8.99

To place an order contact: https://tashai.net

THE IDEAL PROFESSIONAL SPEAKER FOR YOUR NEXT EVENT

Any organization that wants to develop their people to become "extraordinary," needs to hire Tashai for a keynote and/or workshop training!

TO CONTACT OR BOOK TASHAI TO SPEAK:

Tashai Arts LLC
6516 Monona Dr.
Suite 311
Monona, WI 53716

https://tashai.net

THE IDEAL COACH FOR YOU!

If you're ready to overcome challenges, have major breakthroughs, and achieve higher levels, then you will love having Tashai as your coach!

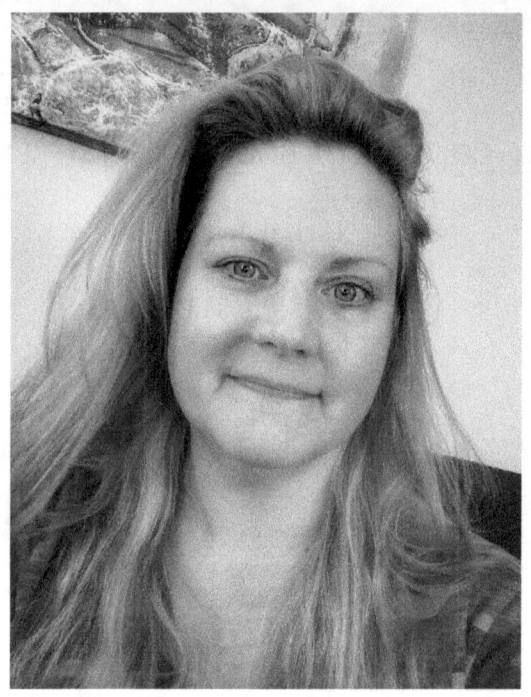

TO CONTACT OR BOOK TASHAI TO SPEAK:
Tashai Arts LLC
6516 Monona Dr. Suite 311
Monona, WI 53716
https://tashai.net

Dedicated to all of you who are striving to live your highest life.

HOW TO USE YOUR TRACKER

Why Should You Bother Creating New Habits of Behavior?

Research has shown that incorporating life-mastering habits—habits designed to propel you forward towards the life you want—is the number one way of becoming more successful. Yet, how do you actually assimilate these new behaviors into your life? How do you turn them into legitimate daily habits? You track them. But of course, having picked up this tracker book, you probably already realize there is something to it.

What are Life-Mastering Habits?

Life-mastering habits are not about worry, struggle or competition. Instead, they are practices that enrich your life, reduce stress, and help align your mental state with the life you've always wanted. Why is this important? Because the powerful principle behind this is simple—if you feel good about yourself, your life will change for the better. Doors will open. Opportunities will arise. And possibilities you can't even fathom right now will materialize. That's how the law of attraction works.

Here are just a few examples that, if done consistently, will bring about the real change you are looking for in your life:

- Meditating
- Exercising
- Reading
- Mind-dump (journaling)
- Visualizing
- Affirmations & Goals
- Tapping (EFT)

In my book, *Fill the Gap: How to Manifest From Where You Are Now to the Life You Want,* (available now on Amazon.com or https://tashai. net) there's an entire chapter on how to integrate life-changing habits into your day. I call it the I AM morning. What does it entail? You simply need to wake up (and get out of bed) one hour earlier than normal. Some people do more, but I encourage you to start with an hour each morning until it truly becomes the norm.

An example from my I AM morning routine is:

- Invigorate (exercise) 20 minutes
- Annotate (journal) 15 minutes
- Meditate (connect) 15 minutes

Invigorate

Do some form of exercise. Walk, run, get on the elliptical or stationary bike, bounce on the rebounder, lift weights, do yoga postures. Find workouts which fit into this time frame and ones that appeal to you. Go at your own pace, and if this is new to you, ease into it. Mix it up too. Changing up your routines on different days will help keep it fresh and will also work different muscles. Be sure to prepare whatever you may need for your workout the night before. This way, there are no excuses not to follow through.

Annotate

Mind-dump journaling. The purpose of this second segment is to clear your head. Get yourself a notebook and write. But there is no specific topic for this kind of journaling. Just write whatever is on your mind, dump it onto the page. Don't worry about sentence structure or grammar, whether it makes sense or not. Dump. You are releasing and opening up space. After a time of doing this, you may find that on some days, insights will come to you. Ideas that might have otherwise escaped your notice will conveniently become clear. Your writing may transform from random thoughts into inspiring messages and exciting new goals. But don't try to make anything happen. Just write whatever comes to you no matter what it is. The goal is to dump.

Meditate

Relax quietly without outside distraction. Meditation is as varied as individuals are. In the beginning, it may help to listen to an audio guided meditation. Or you can focus on a sound, follow your breathing, lay on your back, sit in a chair, or relax in a resting yoga pose. Whatever form of meditation you choose, the purpose here is to connect with your inner self, and it is accomplished by releasing stress and calming the mind. This in turn raises your vibration. Whenever your mind wanders, gently and kindly bring it back to your focal point. Even if you're only able to quiet your mental activity for a brief moment during this time, this will have a sincere impact on the rest of your day. It truly doesn't take much to effect real change.

For more information on meditation, check out my course, *Popping the Bubble: How to Connect With Your Inner Guidance in 7 Days or Less.* https://tashaiarts.samcart.com/products/popping-the-bubble-workshop

Additional Practices

That leaves you 10 minutes to spare in your morning hour. Choose one of the following practices to fill out your session, whichever feels most appropriate for that particular day:

- Visualization
- Tapping (EFT)
- Reading
- Affirmations or goals

Visualization. When you visualize, picture in your mind's eye what it is you would like to achieve or attain. The greater the detail, the more real it becomes for you. Many people use the aid of vision board to which they attach actual photos or magazine clippings of the life they want. Seeing it is important but even more significant is feeling it. When you observe these wonderful images, be sure to also focus on how they make you feel. Bask in it.

Tapping (or Emotional Freedom Technique) is a practice based on the Chinese medicine concept of meridian points found throughout the body. EFT helps clear energetic and emotional blockages, allowing our natural chi (or vital life force) to flow similar to the way that acupuncture and acupressure work. It's easy to learn and involves using your hand to tap points on your head and upper body as you focus on the issue you want to clear, whether it be mental or physical. I devoted a chapter to the tapping process in my previously mentioned book, *Fill the Gap: How to*

Manifest From Where You Are Now to the Life You Want. (on Amazon.com or https://tashai.net)

Read. Take time to read informative, empowering, and uplifting material every week. Read books on health, diet, nature, self-development, financial freedom, universal principles—anything that brings a spark to your life and a spring in your step. Take time to let it in. A well-read individual is an empowered citizen of the world.

Affirmations and goals can be an important and dynamic addition to your life-mastering game plan. I cover these in greater detail below in the section on the *Affirmations & Goals* page.

Of course, if you have some other practice you'd like to substitute, feel free. Whatever calls to you personally is what you want to pursue on a daily basis.

Why Should You Use a Habit Tracker?

Success comes from consistency. The more unfailing you are in your morning practices, the greater the manifestation in the life around you. Studies show that the use of a tracker is an important component in maintaining motivation. It's a visual aid that allows you to see your progress. This, in turn, improves regularity and leads to significant behavior change.

How to Use Your Habit Tracker

An example of the Habit Tracker and how to fill it in can be found at the end of this chapter. Start by circling the month at the top of the page. Then write in the name of each daily practice you are going to track—e.g., meditation, walking, etc. You can see that the days are numbered and run all around the outer edge of the circle.

On day one, after you complete your life-mastering practices, fill in the corresponding space for each with a pencil. I strongly suggest using a different colored pencil for each activity. Yes, it makes it fancy-looking and playful too, however, there is a more significant reason behind this as well. It's subtle but extremely important. Creating a multi-color visual not only makes it easier for you to see your daily progress, it's actually psychologically soothing. It connects your linear thinking mind with your creative emotional side. Accessing both aspects of yourself strengthens your resolve and inspires you to go further.

In addition to the visual incentive of wanting to fill in as many open spaces as possible, you also will be awarding yourself points. Give yourself one point for each time you complete a life-mastering practice. Fill in the box when you reach 90 points. Then again at 120, 140, 160, and 180. Acknowledge yourself each time you do this because these are great accomplishments. Honor yourself for these achievements. At the end of the month, tally up your total points.

What's the prize?

You will decide this before you start each month. Give it some thought. What will you reward yourself if you reach 90 points? And again at 180 points? How will you treat yourself? Make it something fun or exciting for you! Examples could be to go to the beach, take a hike on your favorite trail, do dinner at a nice restaurant, see a new movie or play at the theater, treat yourself to a proffessional shave, facial, or a massage therapy session. Throw a intimate party in your backyard and invite some of your closest friends and the neighbors you've been wanting to meet. Choose whatever feels good to you. Celebrate the progress you are making! You are turning these new habits into your new normal.

What happens if you don't fill in all the spaces or you fall short of your point total? First and foremost, be kind and gentle. Don't berate yourself. This is a process; you are retraining yourself to develop these new habits. This tracker is not about worthiness. You are here, you are alive, you are already worthy and deserving of the life you desire. If there is one thing to take away from all of this, it is that your worthiness is not in question. You belong here! The tracker is simply a tool to help you progress further and further along your path. If you didn't reach your goals this month, simply see if you can up your game in the next one. Maybe the reward you set wasn't enticing enough. If so, try a different one. And if you successfully achieve your goals six months in a row, treat yourself to something extra special. After one year of goals, how about a trip to Disney World—or whatever its equivalent may be for you?

Remember to Care for Yourself Page

Every month you will have a *Remember to Care for Yourself* page. It's easy to get so caught up in reaching your goals that you may forget to live in the moment and be kind to yourself. No hurry, no worry. Take time each and every day to do something nice for yourself. This can be as simple as going outside for a short calming walk. Allowing yourself time for a comfy bubble bath or space in your evening to dive into that book you've been wanting to read for the last year. Filling the diffuser and adding your favorite essential oil scent. Preparing a healthy, delicious meal for yourself. Playing with your cat or dog. Sitting quieting for a few minutes doing absolutely nothing. Or even gazing into your eyes in a mirror and saying aloud that you love and accept yourself exactly as you are. Think simple, think kind, think of yourself.

Make sure you remember to do something nice just for you everyday. Then fill in the star for that day on your page.

Affirmations & Goals Page

Each month, you have four pages (one for each week) to record and review your affirmations and goals. This kind of exercise is highly effective because it focuses your attention in a physical way through the act of writing. It helps to make the statements more real to your subconscious mind. The most effective affirmations and goals are stated in the present tense; in a positive format—i.e., focusing on what you want rather than what you don't want; and with specificity.

In addition, and probably most importantly, is belief. If you have a goal, believe it is possible. It doesn't matter how unrealistic or unattainable it may seem to others. When viewed through the lens of universal principles, quite literally anything is possible. You don't need to know the how, when, or who. You don't have to know anything about it. But you do need to feel the good feeling of what it would be like to have it. If you feel happy when you're daydreaming about it, stay there with that feeling and believe you can have this. Why? Because if you feel it, then there is some aspect of truth in it. It may or may not materialize exactly as you are picturing it right now, but that feeling is an indictor that this is the direction that you should move towards at this point in time.

But what if you want something yet don't really believe you can have it? Step it down a notch or two. Find a goal that still makes you stretch, yet you can also believe in. Bathe in that good feeling until you get to a place where you can transfer that belief to even greater aspirations.

Your goals may remain the same for the entire month, month-to-month, or the whole year. However, it is also just as likely they will change weekly or even daily. As mentioned, you have a page per week to record and update them. Yet, don't hesitate to use additional pieces of paper if needed.

In the act of writing them down, you will find that on some mornings your goals are itching to expand, to shift direction, and synthesize with your new vibration. Pay attention when this happens. It is through the writing that you'll find yourself adjusting words or revising phrases. Fine tune the details and specifics as you grow and change. Write them, review them, write them again.

Your Wins Page

Record your wins for the month. A win is anything that goes your way. A parking spot opens up for you right in front of the grocery store entrance. You get a free side of guacamole for your burrito just because the server was in a good mood. Your kids cleaned their rooms without you having to remind them. An unexpected check comes in the mail. A good friend calls right after you thought about her.

These are all wins, and it's important to recognize and acknowledge them. You created the alignment within yourself which made it possible for these things to occur. The better you feel about yourself, the more aligned you become, and the more the opportunities will come.

So write them down. They can be particularly helpful to look back upon if you are feeling out-of-sorts and need a shot in the arm. The *My Wins* page reminds you just what a bad ass you really are. You're making progress, even when your big bad wolf alter ego is trying its hardest to sucker you into feeling bad.

Your Anything Page

Your Anything Page is for just that, anything. Use it for whatever strikes your fancy, but here are some suggestions:

- Quotes you want to remember
- Potential new ideas
- Messages and inspirations from your higher self
- Vision board pictures
- Relaxing doodles

I sincerely wish you all the success you deserve in life!
Seek happiness and enjoy your journey.

Tashai

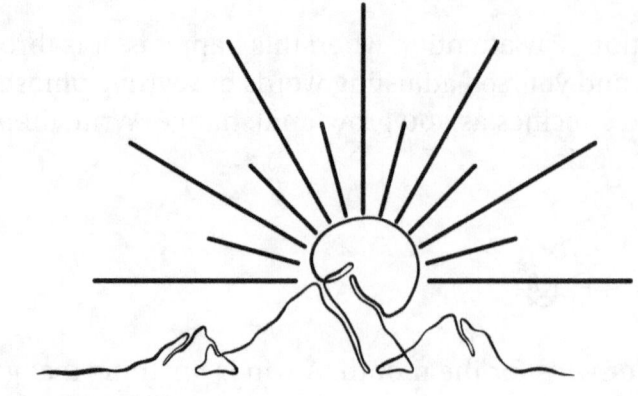

TIPS FOR SUCCESS

- Make sure you set up enticing point rewards for yourself.
- Once you have a few days filled in, you will have visual incentive to keep going.
- Make your tracker as fancy as you want.
- Try colored pencils. They really help!
- Remember this is supposed to be fun!
- Don't hide it! Set this tracker book out where you will see it every day.

HABIT TRACKER - EXAMPLE

MONTH   JAN FEB MAR ~~APR~~ MAY JUN JUL AUG SEPT AUG S EP O CT NOV DEC

write new success habits here

Fill in to track

meditate
annotate
affirmations
tapping
review goals
read
walk

1 2 3 4 5 6 7 8 9 10 11 12 13 14 15 16 17 18 19 20 21 22 23 24 25 26 27 28 29 30 31

Track your points to see how you do each month.
Give your self 1 point for every activity square that you fill in.

90 pts ☐   160 pts ☐   My reward for 90≥
                                    Goto that new place

120 pts ☐   180 pts ☐   *for dinner*

140 pts ☐

My reward for 180≥
                         Get a full body massage

MONTH ONE

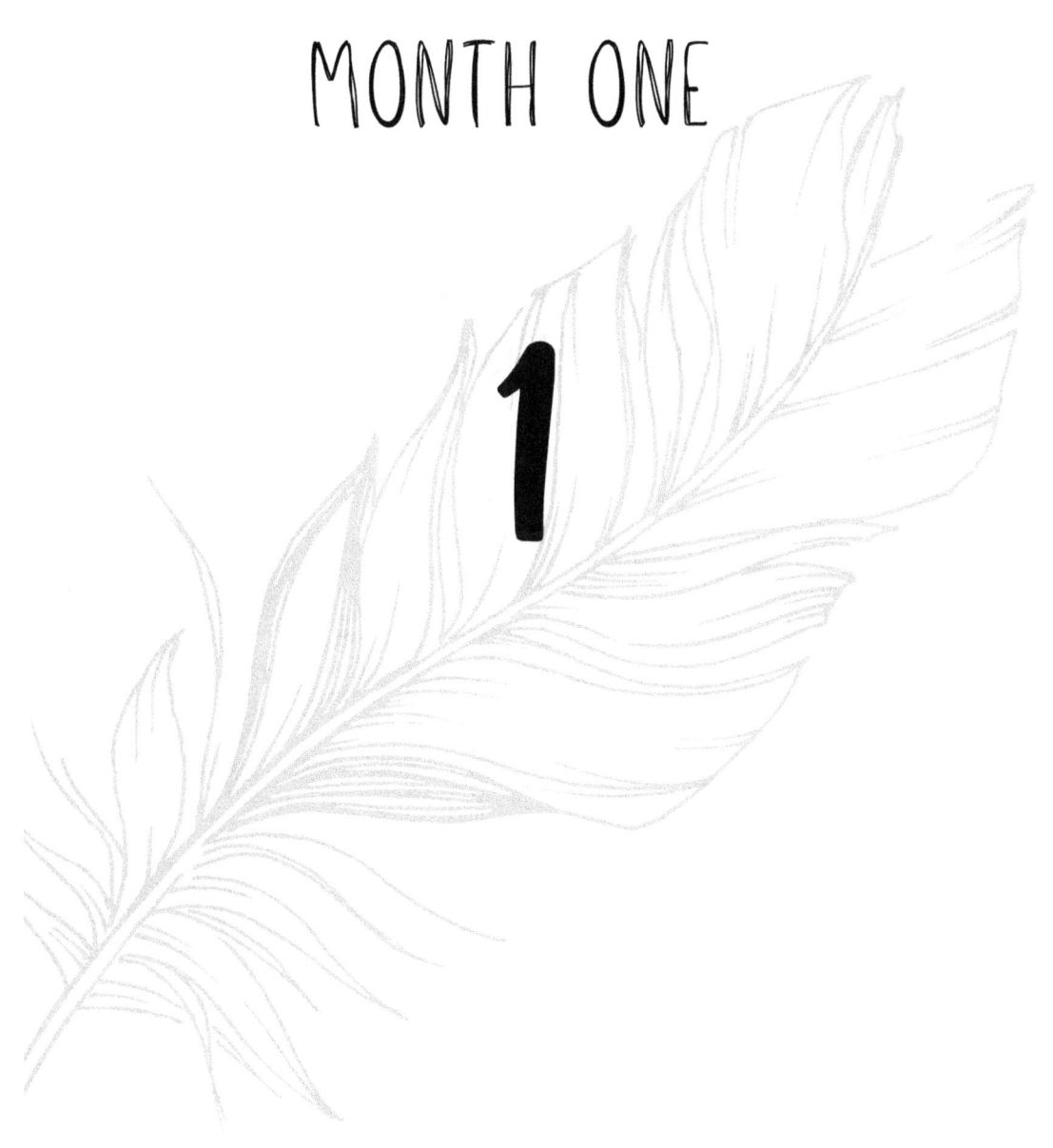

1

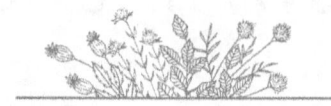

I RELEASE ALL RESISTANCE
AND ALLOW MY NATURAL STATE
OF WELL-BEING TO RISE
TO THE SURFACE.

HABIT TRACKER

MONTH JAN FEB MAR APR MAY JUN JUL AUG SEPT AUG SEP OCT NOV DEC

Track your points to see how you do each month.
Give your self 1 point for every activity square that you fill in.

90 pts ☐   160 pts ☐   My reward for 90≥ _____

120 pts ☐   180 pts ☐   _____

140 pts ☐   My reward for 180≥ _____

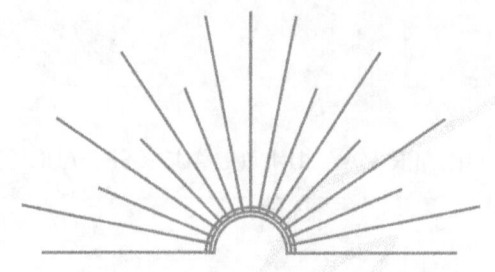

REMEMBER TO CARE FOR YOURSELF

Do something nice for yourself
everyday and fill in a heart

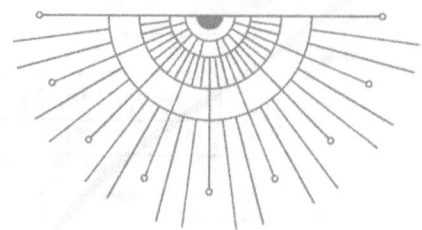

Week 1 - Affirmations / Goals

Week 2 - Affirmations / Goals

Week 3 - Affirmations / Goals

Date :

Week 4 - Affirmations / Goals

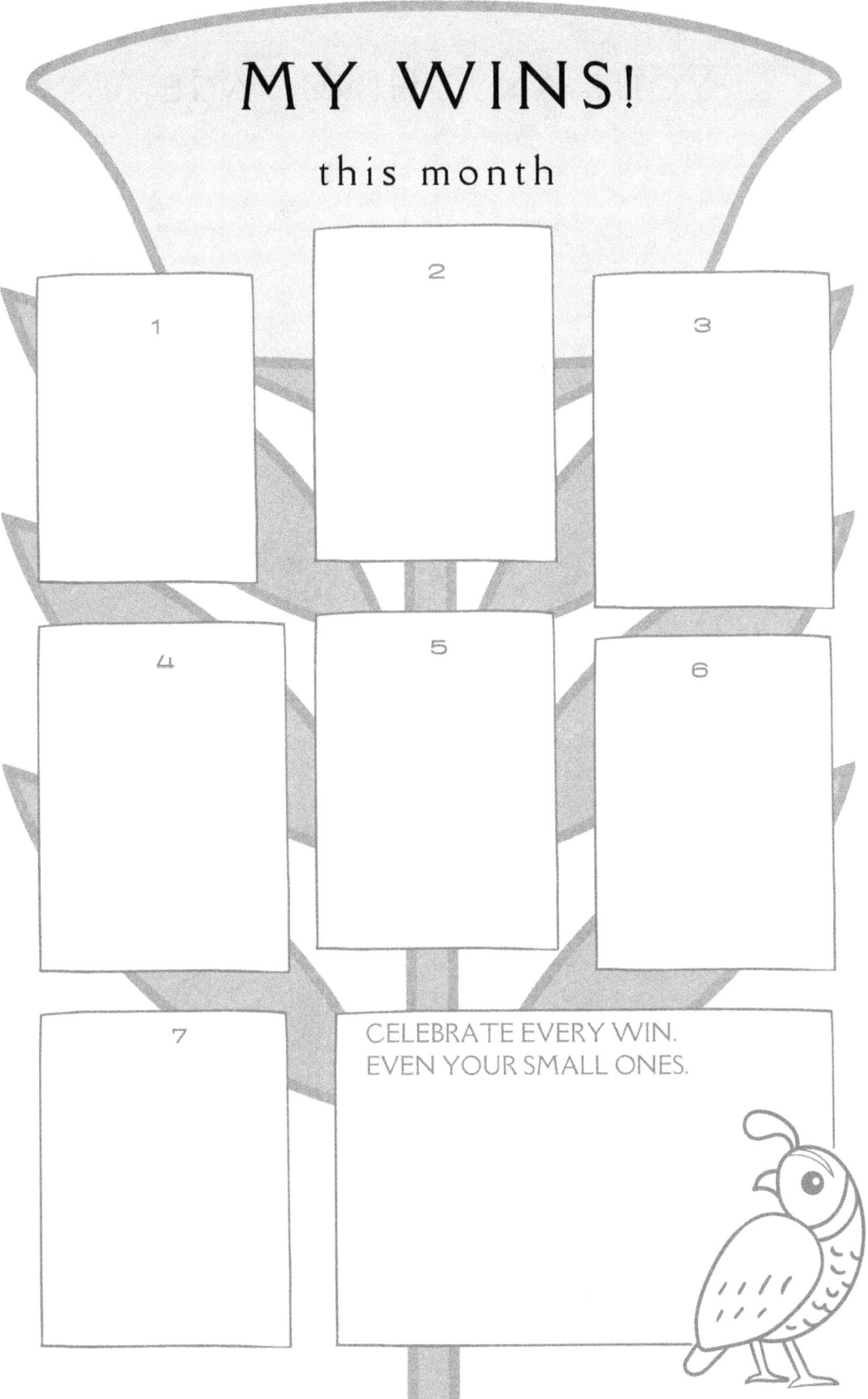

MY WINS!

this month

1

2

3

4

5

6

7

CELEBRATE EVERY WIN.
EVEN YOUR SMALL ONES.

YOUR ANYTHING PAGE

YOUR ANYTHING PAGE

"OPPORTUNITY IS MISSED BY MOST PEOPLE BECAUSE IT IS DRESSED IN OVERALLS AND LOOKS LIKE WORK." — THOMAS EDISON

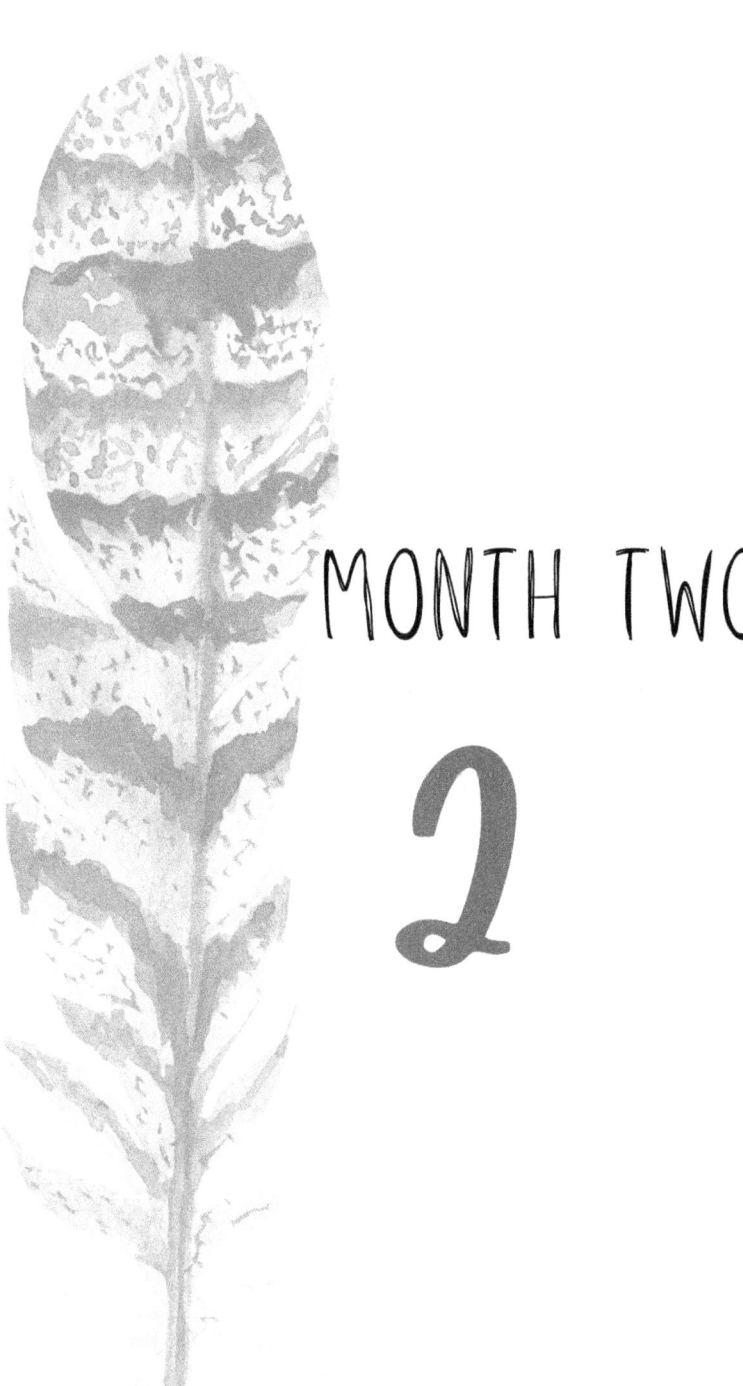

MONTH TWO

2

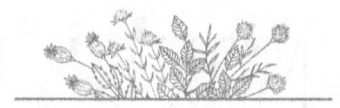

I TAKE 100% RESPONSIBILITY
FOR EVERYTHING IN MY LIFE.

HABIT TRACKER

MONTH JAN FEB MAR APR MAY JUN JUL AUG SEPT AUG SEP OCT NOV DEC

Track your points to see how you do each month.
Give your self 1 point for every activity square that you fill in.

90 pts ☐   160 pts ☐   My reward for 90≥ _____

120 pts ☐   180 pts ☐   _____

140 pts ☐   My reward for 180≥ _____

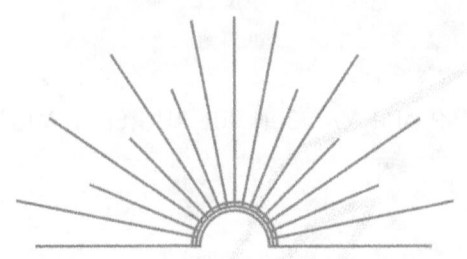

REMEMBER TO CARE FOR YOURSELF

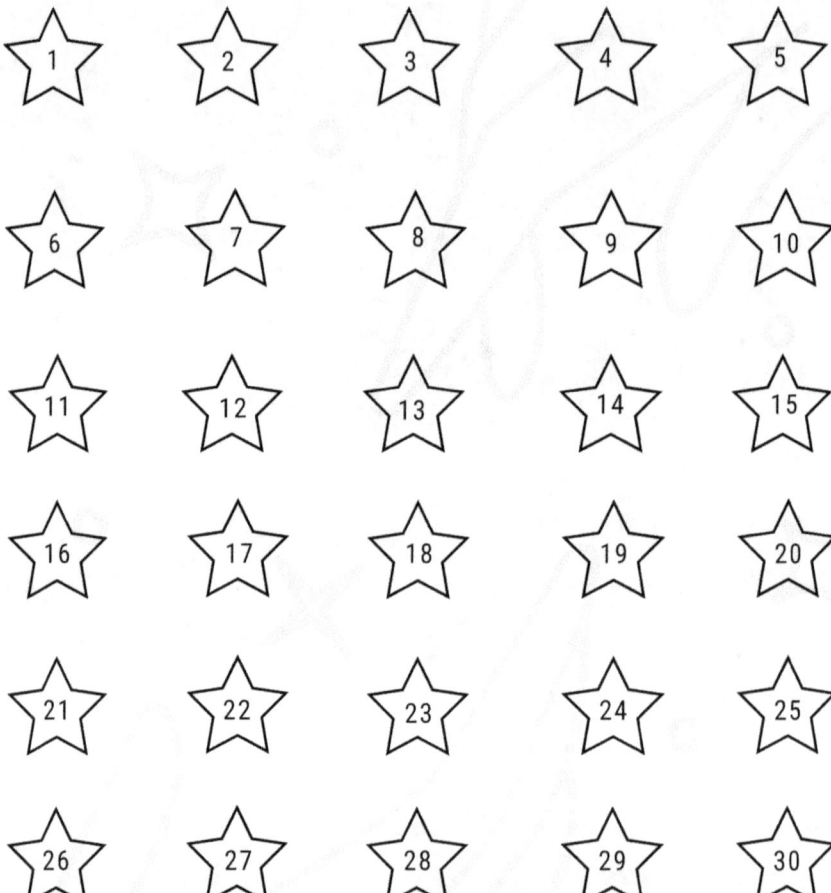

1 2 3 4 5

6 7 8 9 10

11 12 13 14 15

16 17 18 19 20

21 22 23 24 25

26 27 28 29 30

31 Do something nice for yourself
everyday and fill in a heart

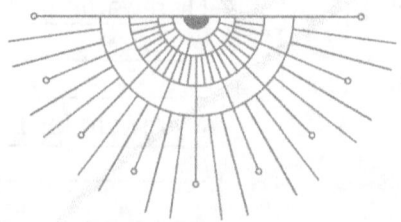

Week 1 - Affirmations / Goals

Date :

Week 2 - Affirmations / Goals

Week 3 - Affirmations / Goals

Week 4 - Affirmations / Goals   Date :

MY WINS!

this month

1

2

3

4

5

6

7

CELEBRATE EVERY WIN.
EVEN YOUR SMALL ONES.

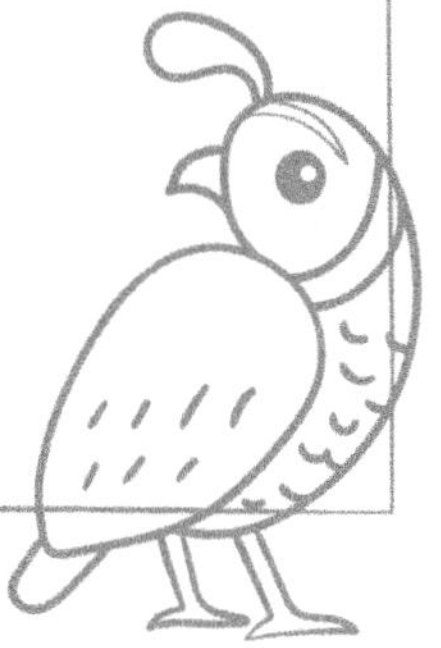

YOUR ANYTHING PAGE

"ANYTHING WORTH HAVING TAKES TIME"

YOUR ANYTHING PAGE

DATE:

MONTH THREE

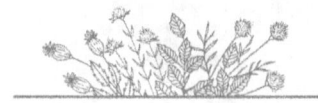

I ATTRACT THE RIGHT PEOPLE,
CIRCUMSTANCES, AND EVENTS TO
HELP ME MOVE JOYOUSLY
FORWARD ALONG MY PATH.

HABIT TRACKER

MONTH   JAN FEB MAR APR MAY JUN JUL AUG SEPT AUG SEP OCT NOV DEC

Track your points to see how you do each month.
Give your self 1 point for every activity square that you fill in.

90 pts	☐	160 pts	☐	My reward for 90≥
120 pts	☐	180 pts	☐	
140 pts	☐			My reward for 180≥

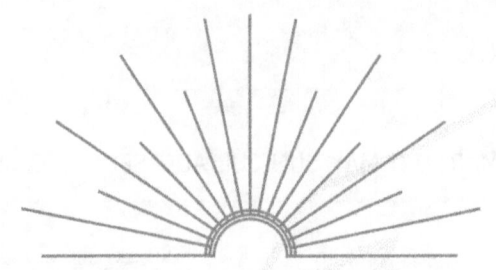

REMEMBER TO CARE FOR YOURSELF

Do something nice for yourself
everyday and fill in a heart

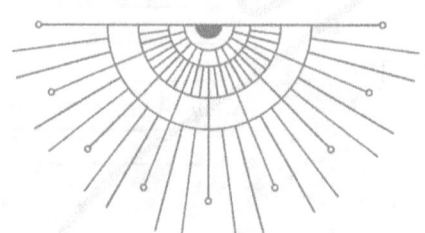

Week 1 - Affirmations / Goals

Week 2 - Affirmations / Goals

Week 3 - Affirmations / Goals

Week 4 - Affirmations / Goals   Date :

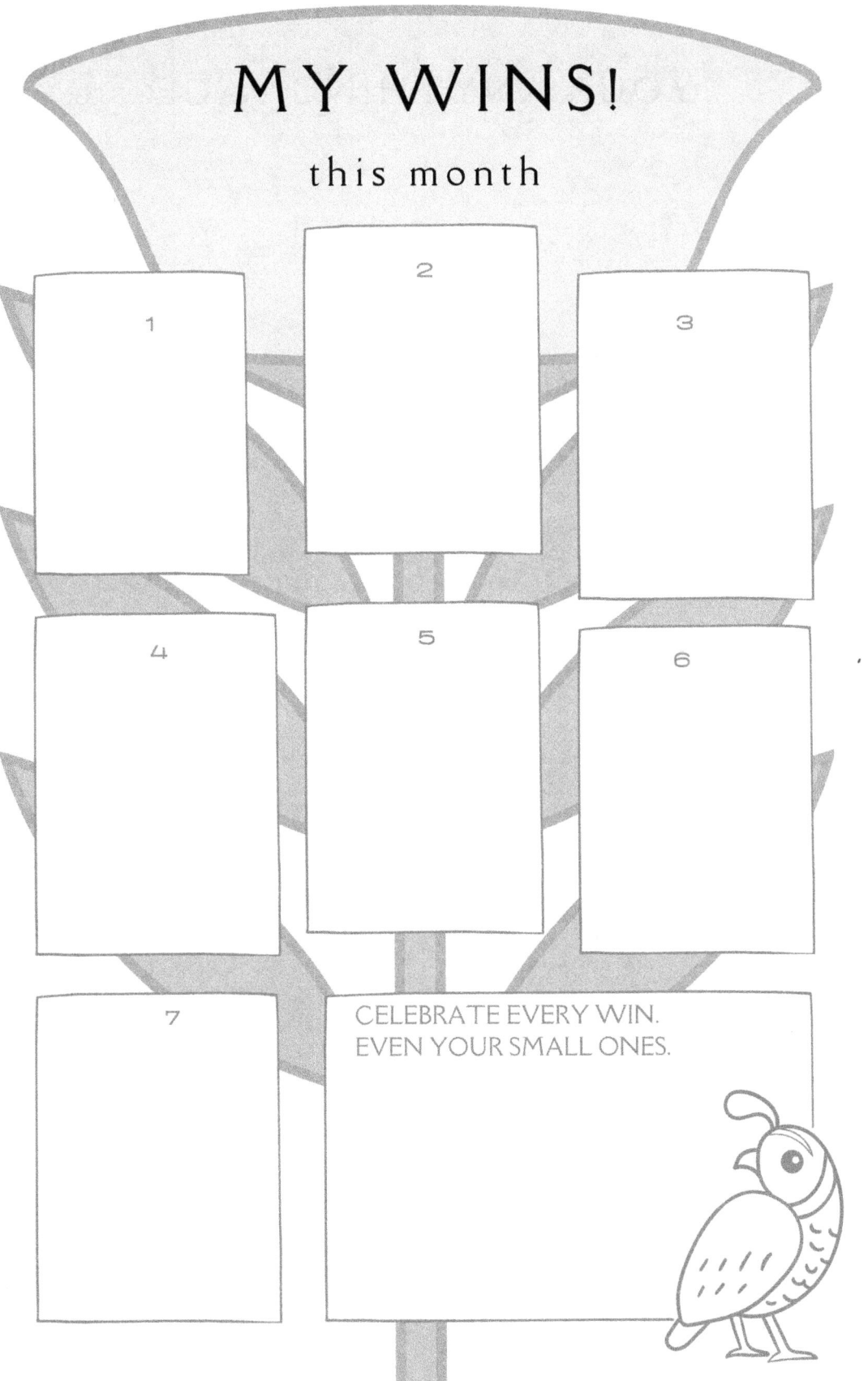

MY WINS!

this month

1

2

3

4

5

6

7

CELEBRATE EVERY WIN.
EVEN YOUR SMALL ONES.

YOUR ANYTHING PAGE

DATE:

YOUR ANYTHING PAGE

MONTH FOUR

4

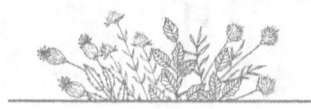

I HAVE A LIFE OF
EASE, INSPIRATION,
AND PROSPERITY.

HABIT TRACKER

MONTH JAN FEB MAR APR MAY JUN JUL AUG SEPT AUG SEP OCT NOV DEC

Track your points to see how you do each month.
Give your self 1 point for every activity square that you fill in.

90 pts ☐   160 pts ☐   My reward for 90≥ _____

120 pts ☐   180 pts ☐   _____

140 pts ☐   My reward for 180≥ _____

_____

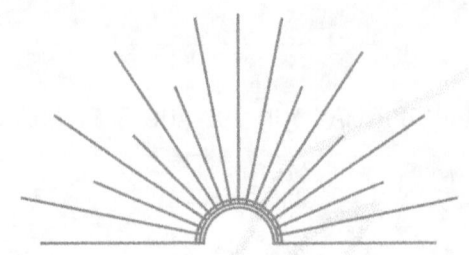

REMEMBER TO CARE FOR YOURSELF

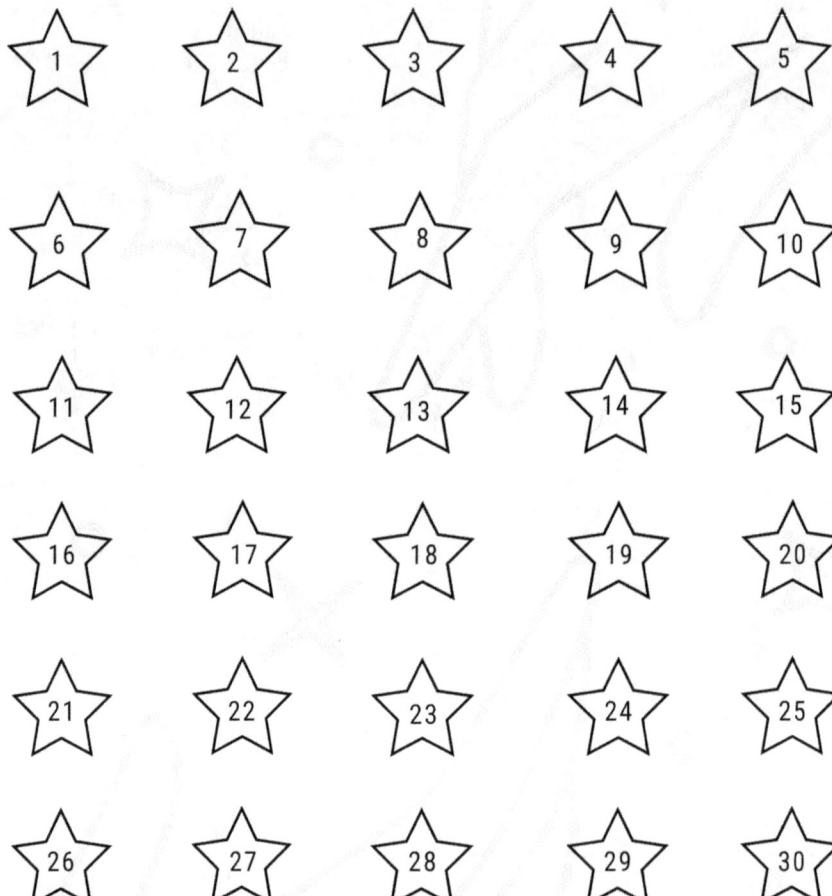

1 2 3 4 5

6 7 8 9 10

11 12 13 14 15

16 17 18 19 20

21 22 23 24 25

26 27 28 29 30

31

Do something nice for yourself
everyday and fill in a heart

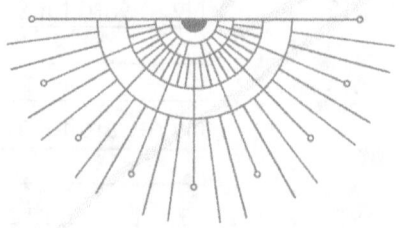

Week 1 - Affirmations / Goals

Week 2 - Affirmations / Goals

Week 3 - Affirmations / Goals

Week 4 - Affirmations / Goals   Date :

MY WINS!

this month

1

2

3

4

5

6

7

CELEBRATE EVERY WIN.
EVEN YOUR SMALL ONES.

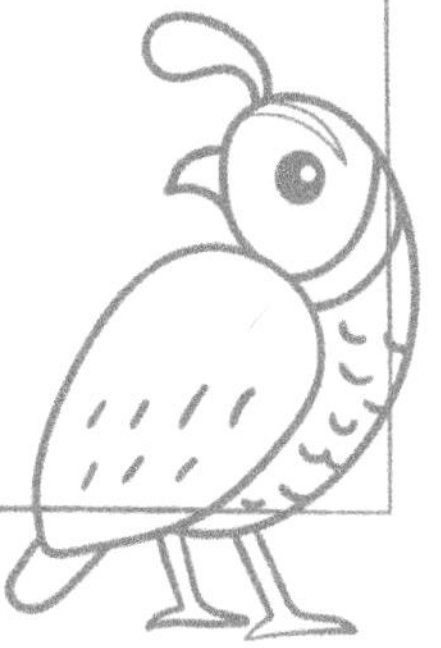

YOUR ANYTHING PAGE

YOUR ANYTHING PAGE

"JOURNALING IS LIKE WHISPERING TO ONE'S SELF AND LISTENING
AT THE SAME TIME." – MINA MURRAY, DRACULA

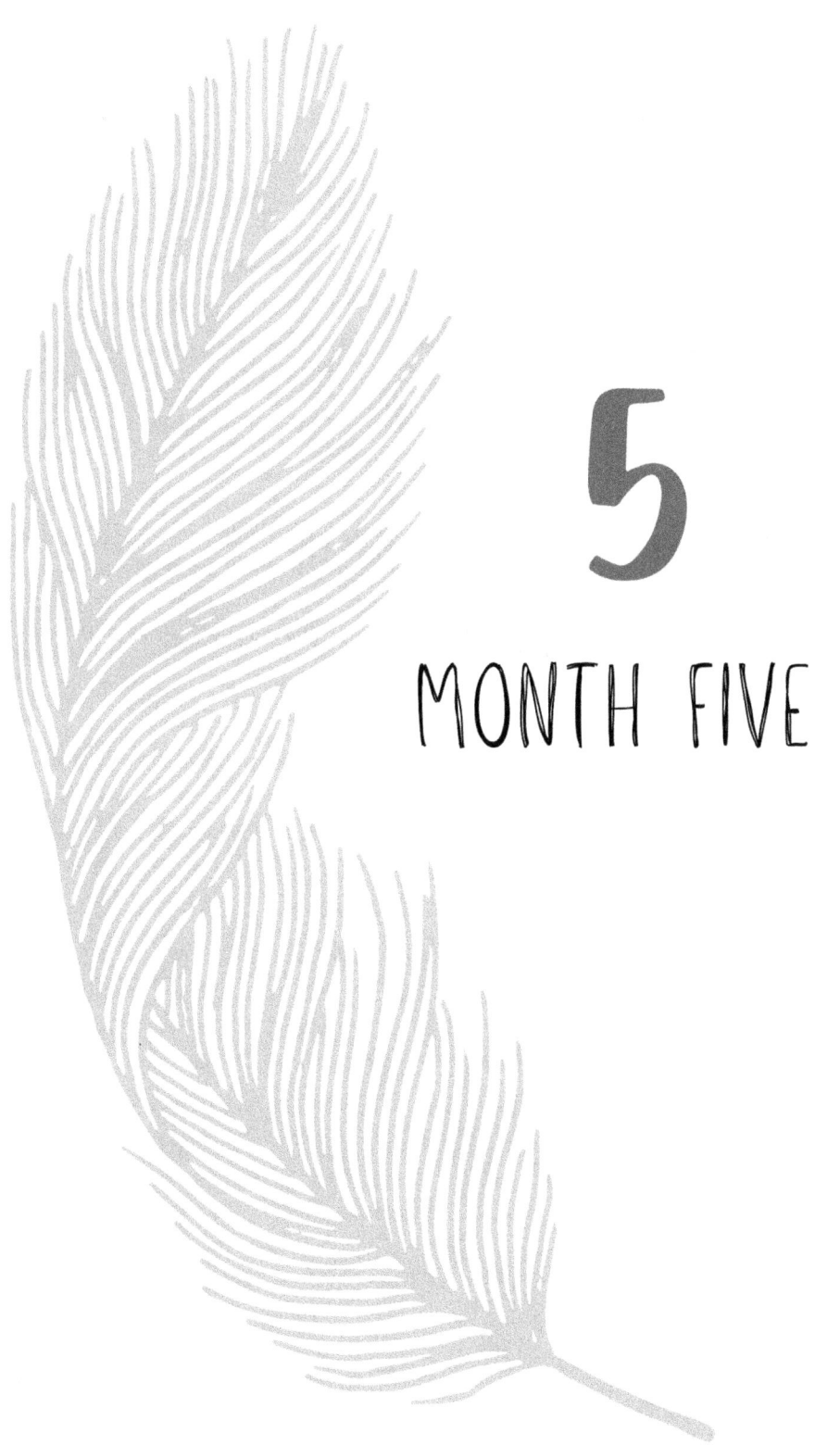

5

MONTH FIVE

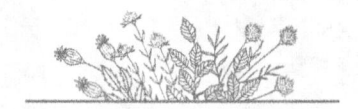

I ALWAYS SHOW UP
FOR MYSELF.

HABIT TRACKER

MONTH   JAN FEB MAR APR MAY JUN JUL AUG SEPT AUG SEP OCT NOV DEC

Track your points to see how you do each month.
Give your self 1 point for every activity square that you fill in.

90 pts ☐   160 pts ☐   My reward for 90≥ _____

120 pts ☐   180 pts ☐   _____

140 pts ☐   My reward for 180≥ _____

_____

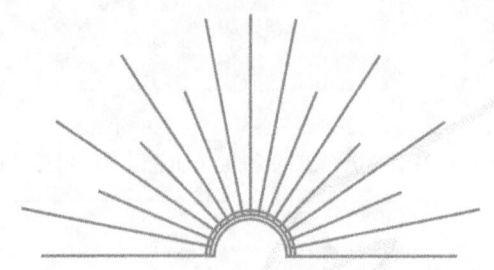

REMEMBER TO CARE FOR YOURSELF

 Do something nice for yourself
everyday and fill in a heart

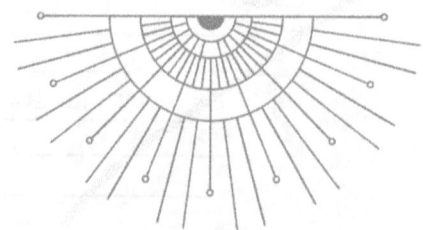

Week 1 - Affirmations / Goals

Date :

Week 2 - Affirmations / Goals

Week 3 - Affirmations / Goals

Week 4 - Affirmations / Goals

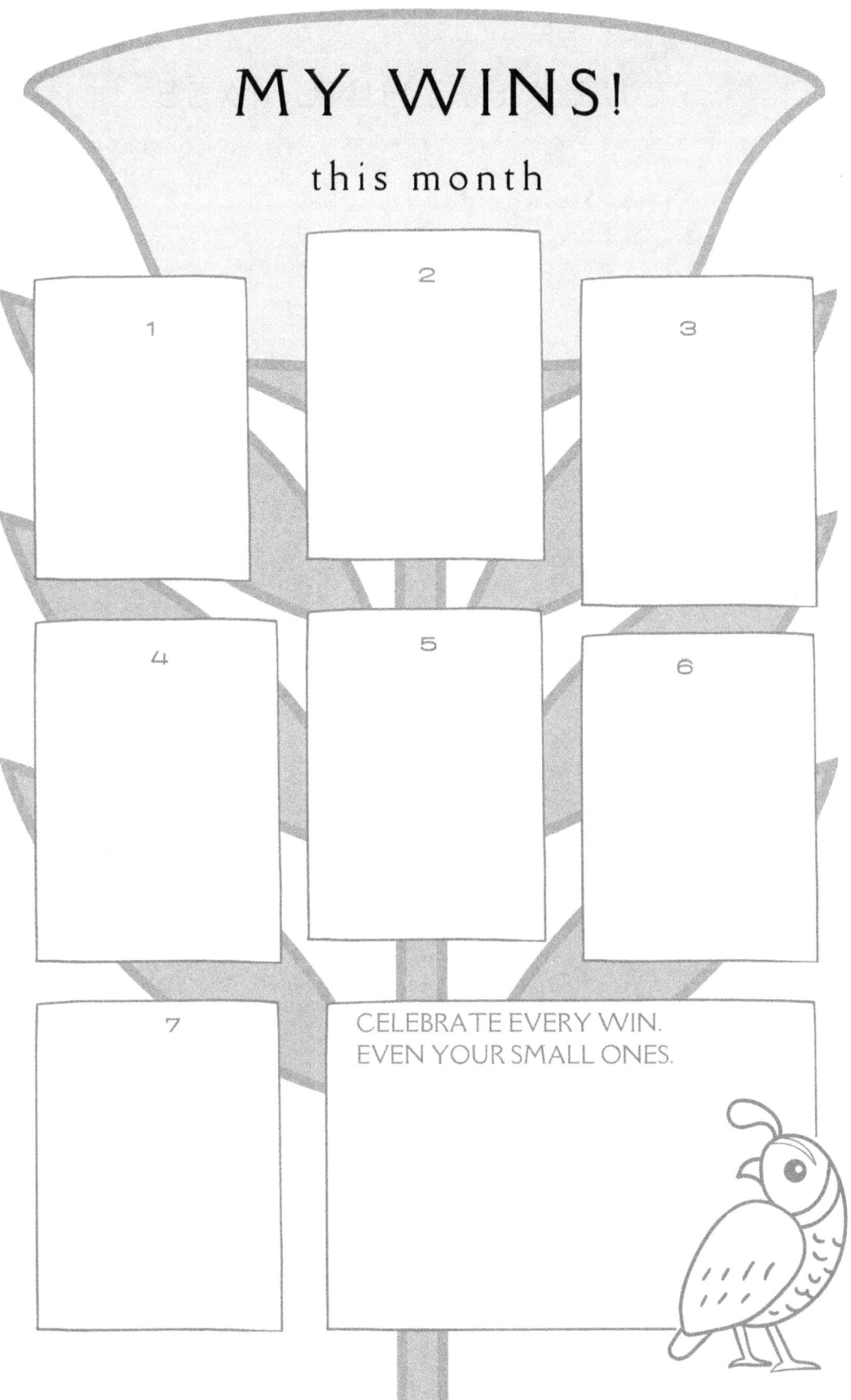

MY WINS!

this month

1

2

3

4

5

6

7

CELEBRATE EVERY WIN.
EVEN YOUR SMALL ONES.

YOUR ANYTHING PAGE

DATE:

YOUR ANYTHING PAGE

"WRITING IS MEDICINE. IT IS AN APPROPRIATE ANTIDOTE TO INJURY.
IT IS AN APPROPRIATE COMPANION FOR ANY DIFFICULT CHANGE."
—JULIA CAMERON

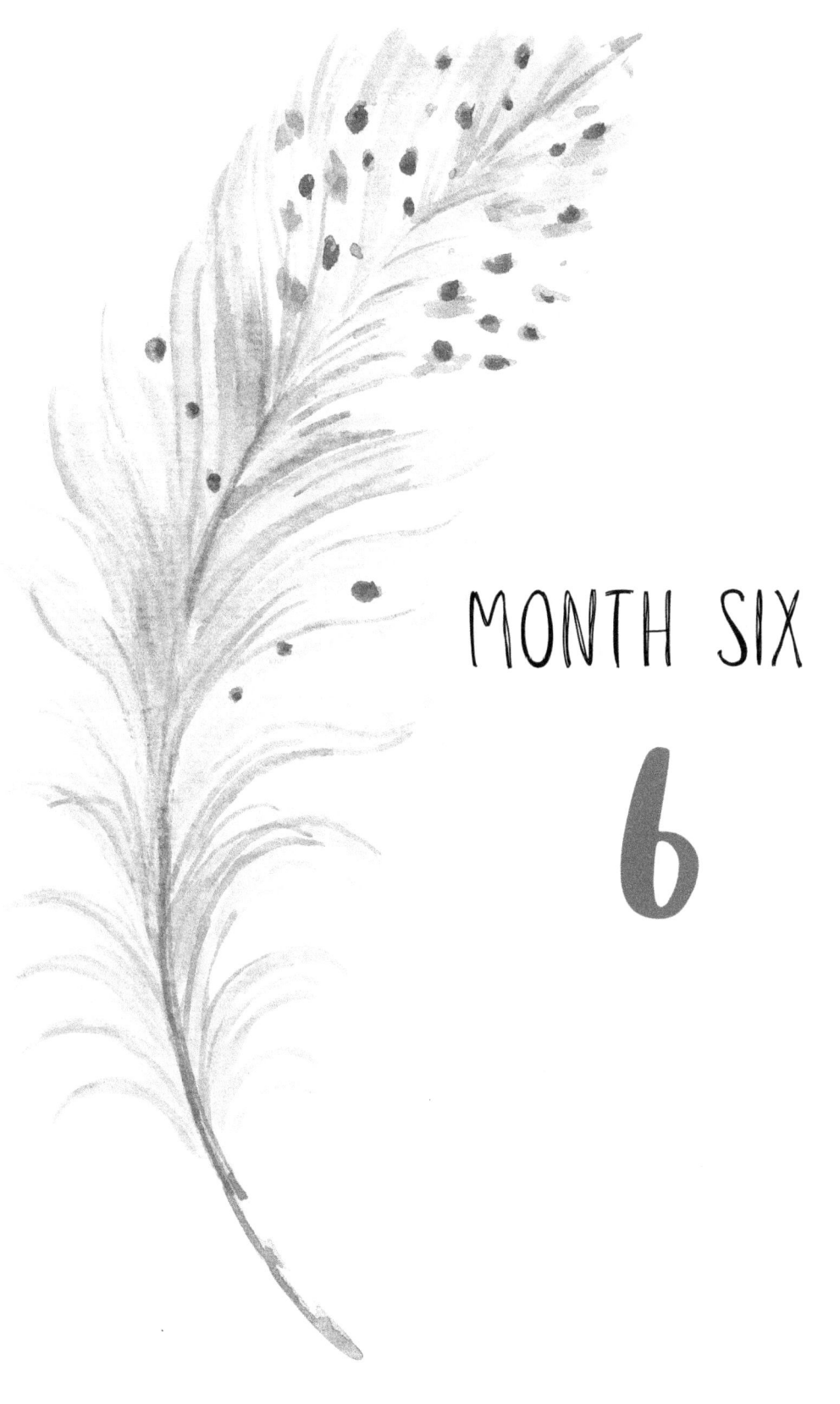

MONTH SIX

6

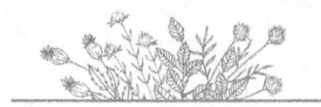

THE SOURCE OF WHO
I REALLY AM IS
LOVE AND JOY.

HABIT TRACKER

MONTH JAN FEB MAR APR MAY JUN JUL AUG SEPT AUG SEP OCT NOV DEC

Track your points to see how you do each month.
Give your self 1 point for every activity square that you fill in.

90 pts ☐   160 pts ☐   My reward for 90≥ _____

120 pts ☐   180 pts ☐   _____

140 pts ☐   My reward for 180≥ _____

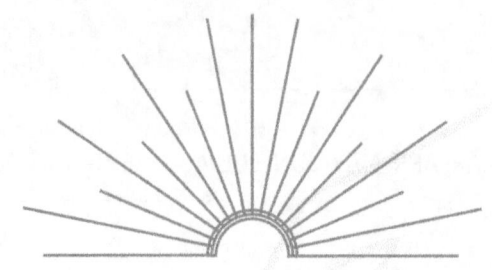

REMEMBER TO CARE FOR YOURSELF

 1    2    3    4    5

 6    7    8    9    10

 11    12    13    14    15

 16    17    18    19    20

 21    22    23    24    25

 26    27    28    29    30

 31   Do something nice for yourself everyday and fill in a heart

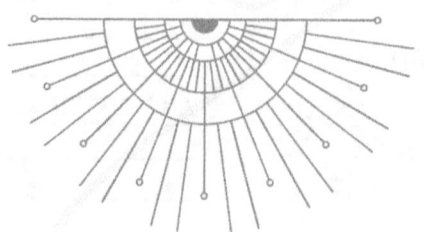

Week 1 - Affirmations / Goals

Week 2 - Affirmations / Goals

Week 3 - Affirmations / Goals

Week 4 - Affirmations / Goals

Date :

MY WINS!

this month

1

2

3

4

5

6

7

CELEBRATE EVERY WIN.
EVEN YOUR SMALL ONES.

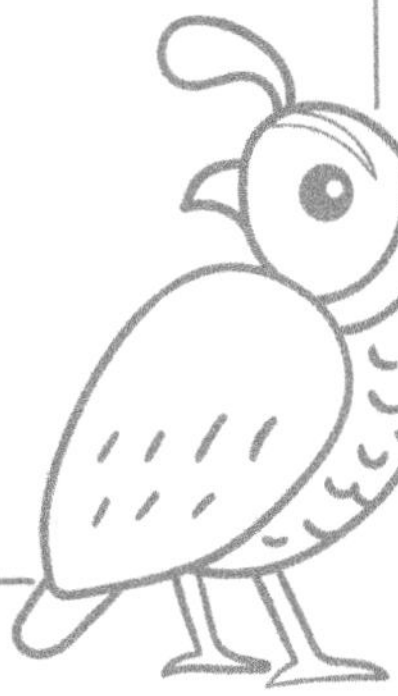

YOUR ANYTHING PAGE

DATE:

YOUR ANYTHING PAGE

"WRITE WHAT DISTURBS YOU, WHAT YOU FEAR, WHAT YOU HAVE NOT BEEN WILLING TO SPEAK ABOUT. BE WILLING TO BE SPLIT OPEN." —NATALIE GOLDBERG

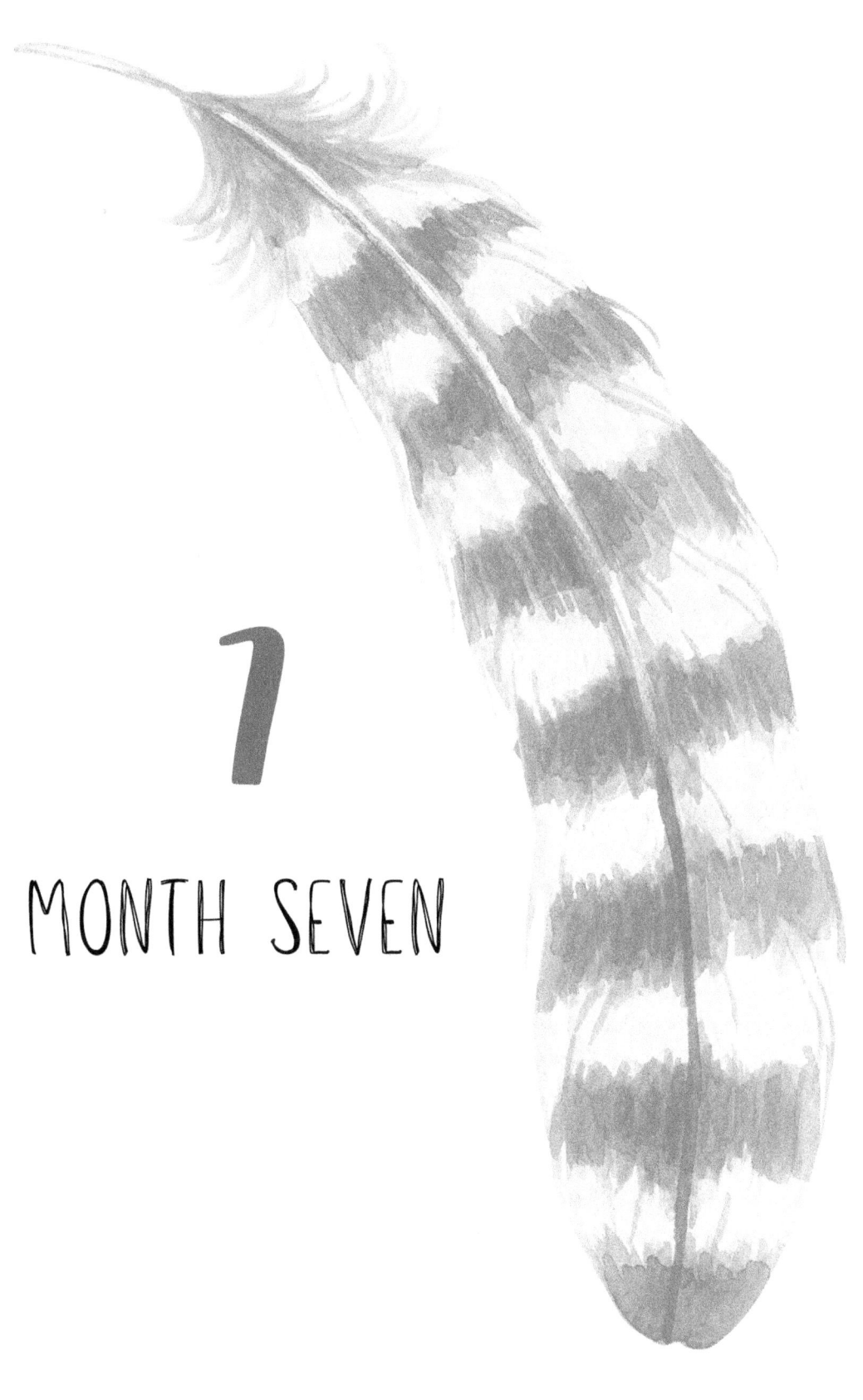

1

MONTH SEVEN

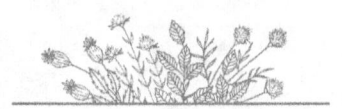

I AM MANIFESTING
NEW OPPORTUNITIES
ALL THE TIME.

HABIT TRACKER

MONTH JAN FEB MAR APR MAY JUN JUL AUG SEPT AUG SEP OCT NOV DEC

Track your points to see how you do each month.
Give your self 1 point for every activity square that you fill in.

90 pts	☐	160 pts	☐
120 pts	☐	180 pts	☐
140 pts	☐		

My reward for 90≥ _____

_____

My reward for 180≥ _____

_____

_____

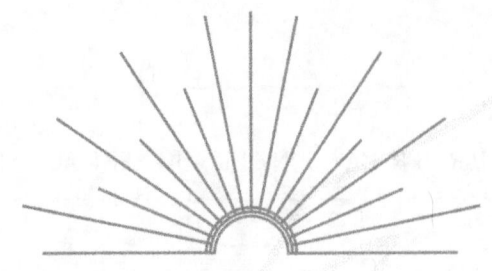

REMEMBER TO CARE FOR YOURSELF

 1    2    3    4    5

 6    7    8    9    10

 11    12    13    14    15

 16    17    18    19    20

 21    22    23    24    25

 26    27    28    29    30

 31   Do something nice for yourself everyday and fill in a heart

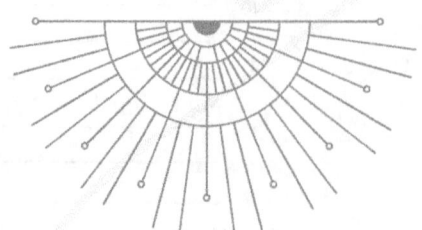

Week 1 - Affirmations / Goals

Week 2 - Affirmations / Goals

Date :

Week 3 - Affirmations / Goals

Week 4 - Affirmations / Goals

Date :

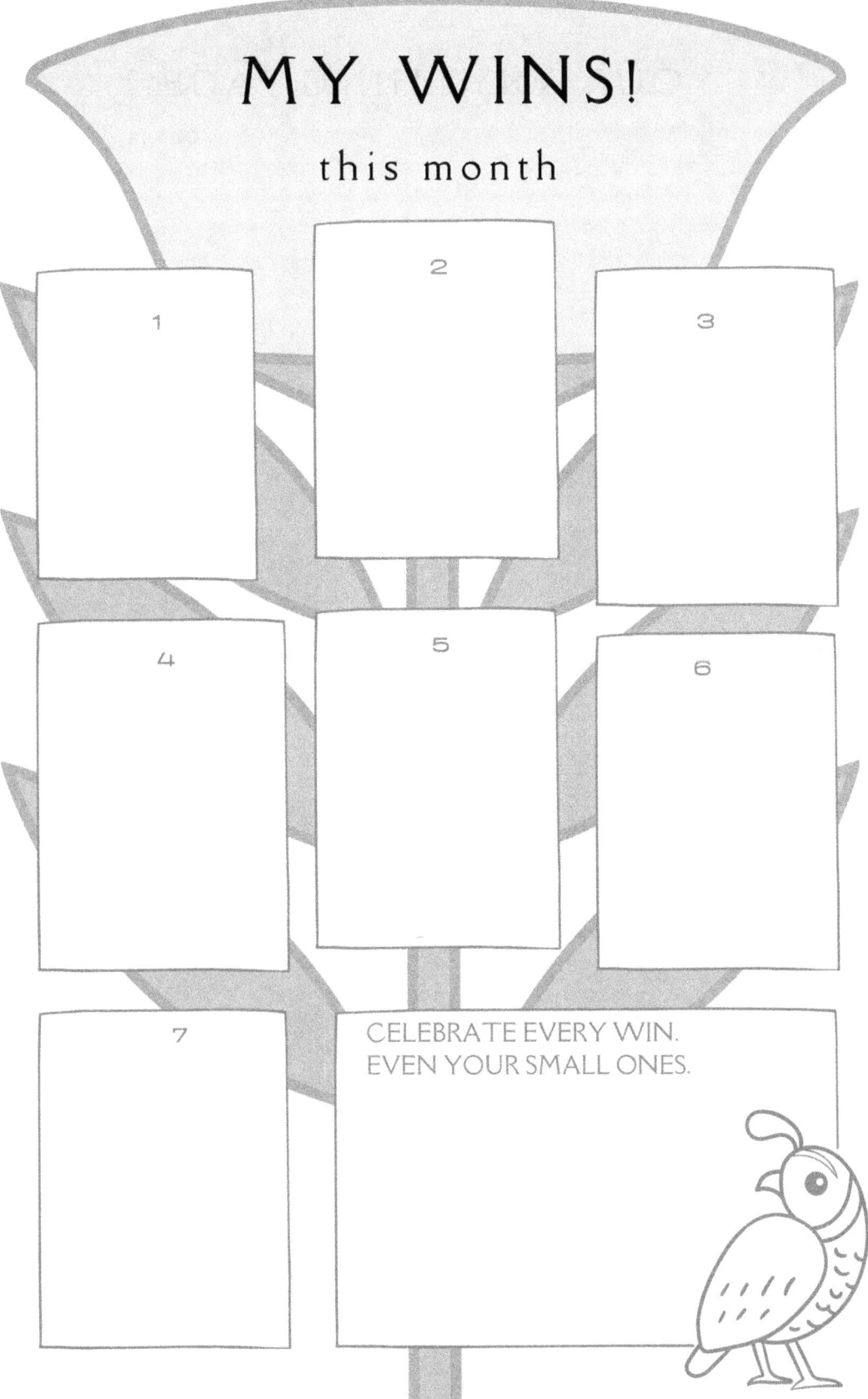

MY WINS!
this month

1

2

3

4

5

6

7

CELEBRATE EVERY WIN.
EVEN YOUR SMALL ONES.

YOUR ANYTHING PAGE

"JOURNAL WRITING IS A VOYAGE TO THE INTERIOR."
—CHRISTINA BALDWIN

YOUR ANYTHING PAGE

"KEEPING A JOURNAL OF WHAT'S GOING ON IN YOUR LIFE IS A GOOD
WAY TO HELP YOU DISTILL WHAT'S IMPORTANT AND WHAT'S NOT."
—MARTINA NAVRATILOVA

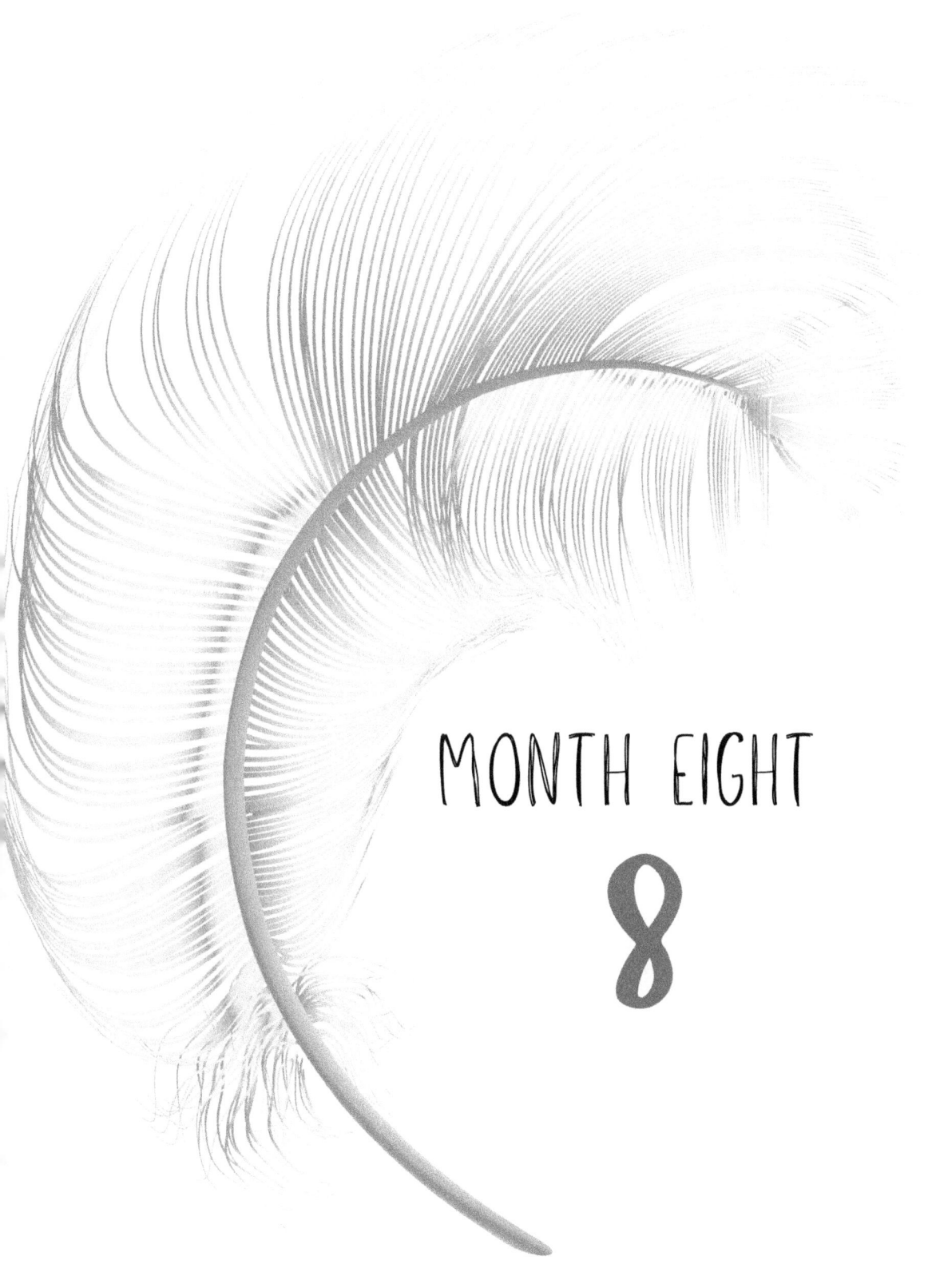

MONTH EIGHT

8

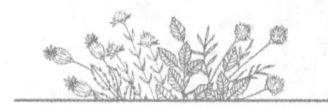

I ALWAYS MOVE IN THE
DIRECTION OF MY HIGHER KNOWING
AND LIFE UNFOLDS IN
MAGNIFICENT WAYS.

HABIT TRACKER

MONTH JAN FEB MAR APR MAY JUN JUL AUG SEPT AUG SEP OCT NOV DEC

Track your points to see how you do each month.
Give your self 1 point for every activity square that you fill in.

90 pts ☐ 160 pts ☐ My reward for 90≥ _____

120 pts ☐ 180 pts ☐ _____

140 pts ☐ My reward for 180≥ _____

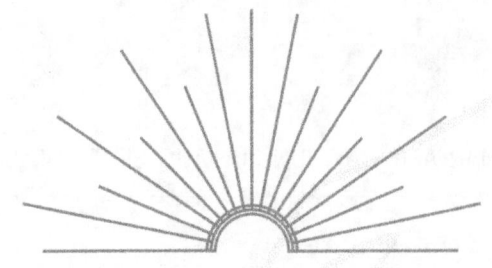

REMEMBER TO CARE FOR YOURSELF

Do something nice for yourself
everyday and fill in a heart

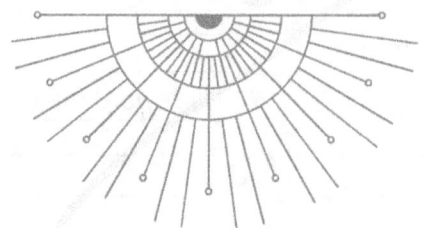

Week 1 - Affirmations / Goals

Date :

Week 2 - Affirmations / Goals

Week 3 - Affirmations / Goals

Week 4 - Affirmations / Goals

MY WINS!

this month

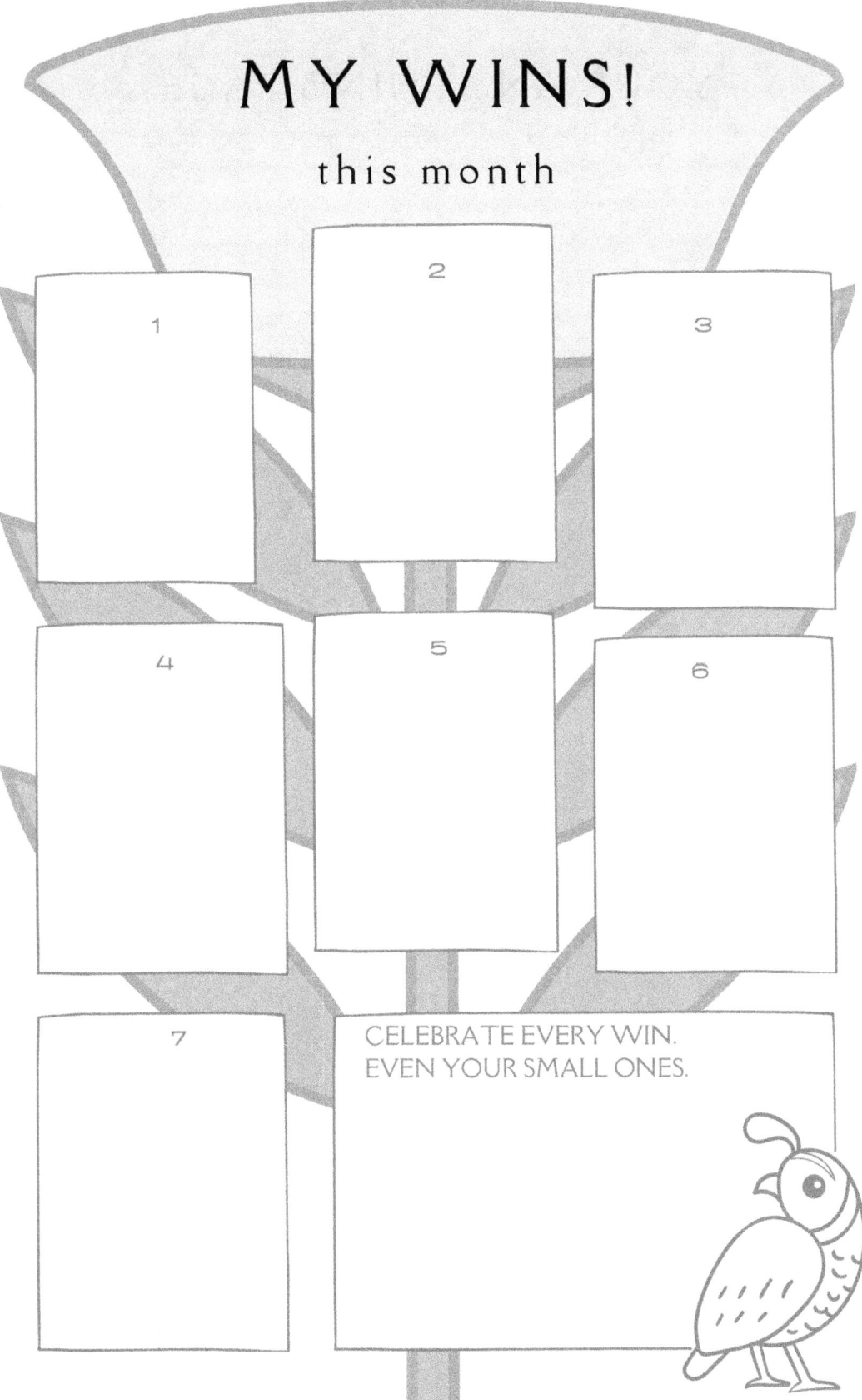

1

2

3

4

5

6

7

CELEBRATE EVERY WIN.
EVEN YOUR SMALL ONES.

YOUR ANYTHING PAGE

YOUR ANYTHING PAGE

DATE:

MONTH NINE

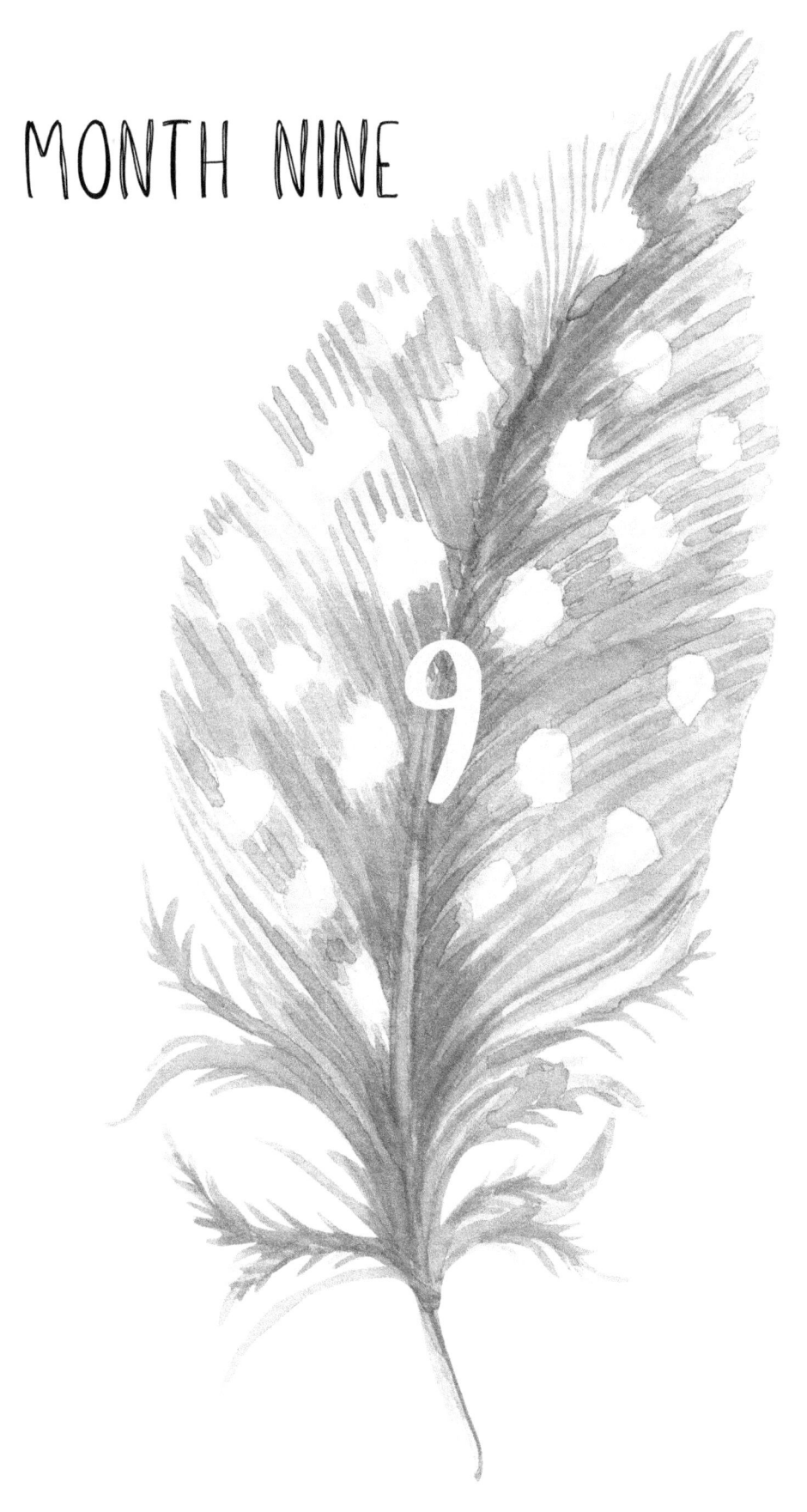

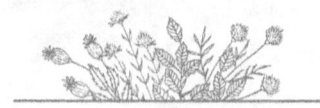

I GENTLY TUNE MY THOUGHTS
WITH THE THINGS THAT
BRING ME JOY.

HABIT TRACKER

MONTH JAN FEB MAR APR MAY JUN JUL AUG SEPT AUG SEP OCT NOV DEC

Track your points to see how you do each month.
Give your self 1 point for every activity square that you fill in.

90 pts ☐   160 pts ☐   My reward for 90≥ _____

120 pts ☐   180 pts ☐   _____

140 pts ☐   My reward for 180≥ _____

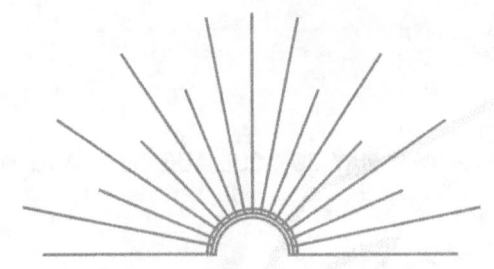

REMEMBER TO CARE FOR YOURSELF

 1  2  3  4  5

 6  7  8  9  10

 11  12  13  14  15

 16  17  18  19  20

 21  22  23  24  25

 26  27  28  29  30

 31

Do something nice for yourself
everyday and fill in a heart

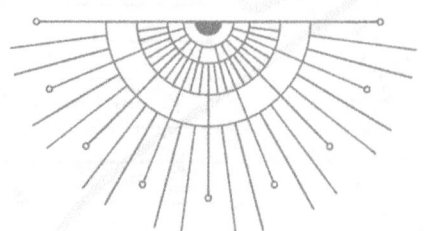

Week 1 - Affirmations / Goals

Week 2 - Affirmations / Goals

Date :

Week 3 - Affirmations / Goals

Date :

Week 4 - Affirmations / Goals

Date :

MY WINS!

this month

1

2

3

4

5

6

7

CELEBRATE EVERY WIN.
EVEN YOUR SMALL ONES.

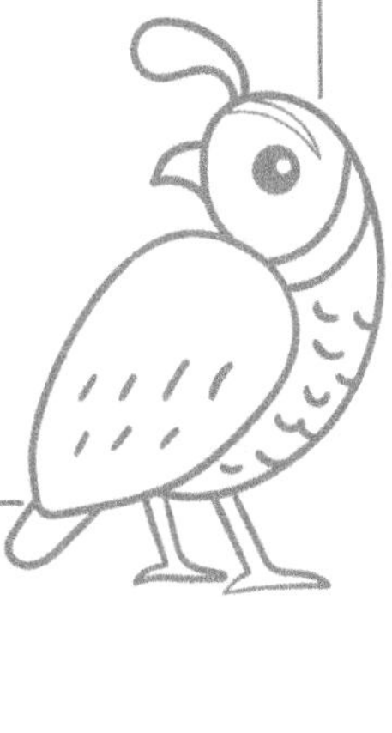

YOUR ANYTHING PAGE

YOUR ANYTHING PAGE

DATE:

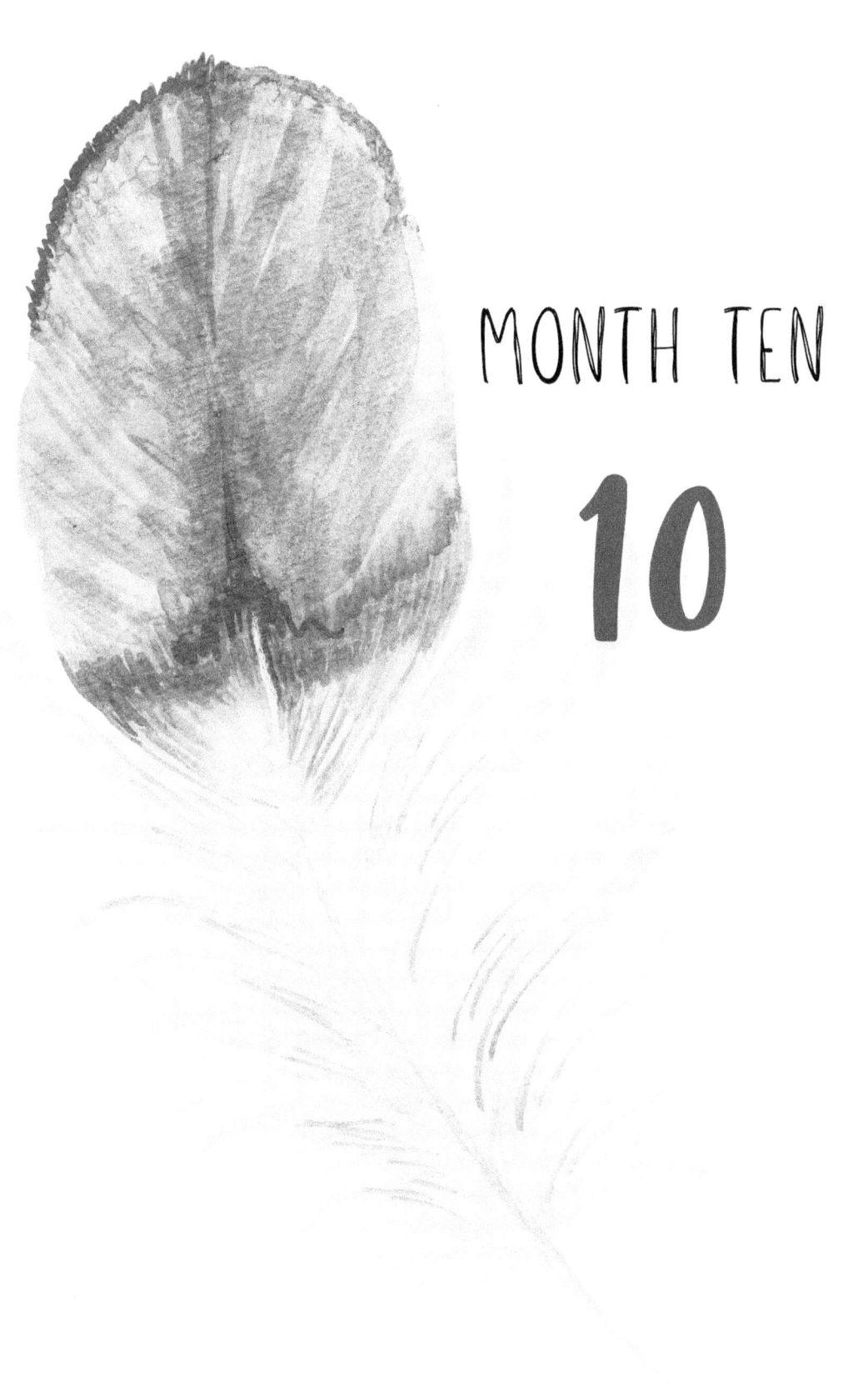

MONTH TEN

10

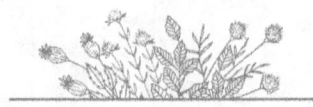

MY INNER BEING IS CALLING
ME FORWARD TO THE
LIFE I WANT.

HABIT TRACKER

MONTH JAN FEB MAR APR MAY JUN JUL AUG SEPT AUG SEP OCT NOV DEC

Track your points to see how you do each month.
Give your self 1 point for every activity square that you fill in.

90 pts	☐	160 pts	☐	My reward for 90≥ _____
120 pts	☐	180 pts	☐	_____
140 pts	☐			My reward for 180≥ _____

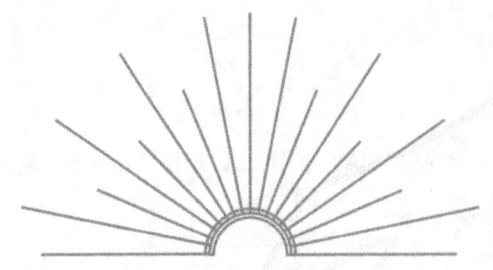

REMEMBER TO CARE FOR YOURSELF

 Do something nice for yourself
everyday and fill in a heart

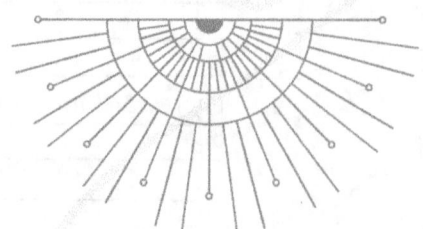

Week 1 - Affirmations / Goals

Date :

Week 2 - Affirmations / Goals

Week 3 - Affirmations / Goals   Date :

Week 4 - Affirmations / Goals   Date :

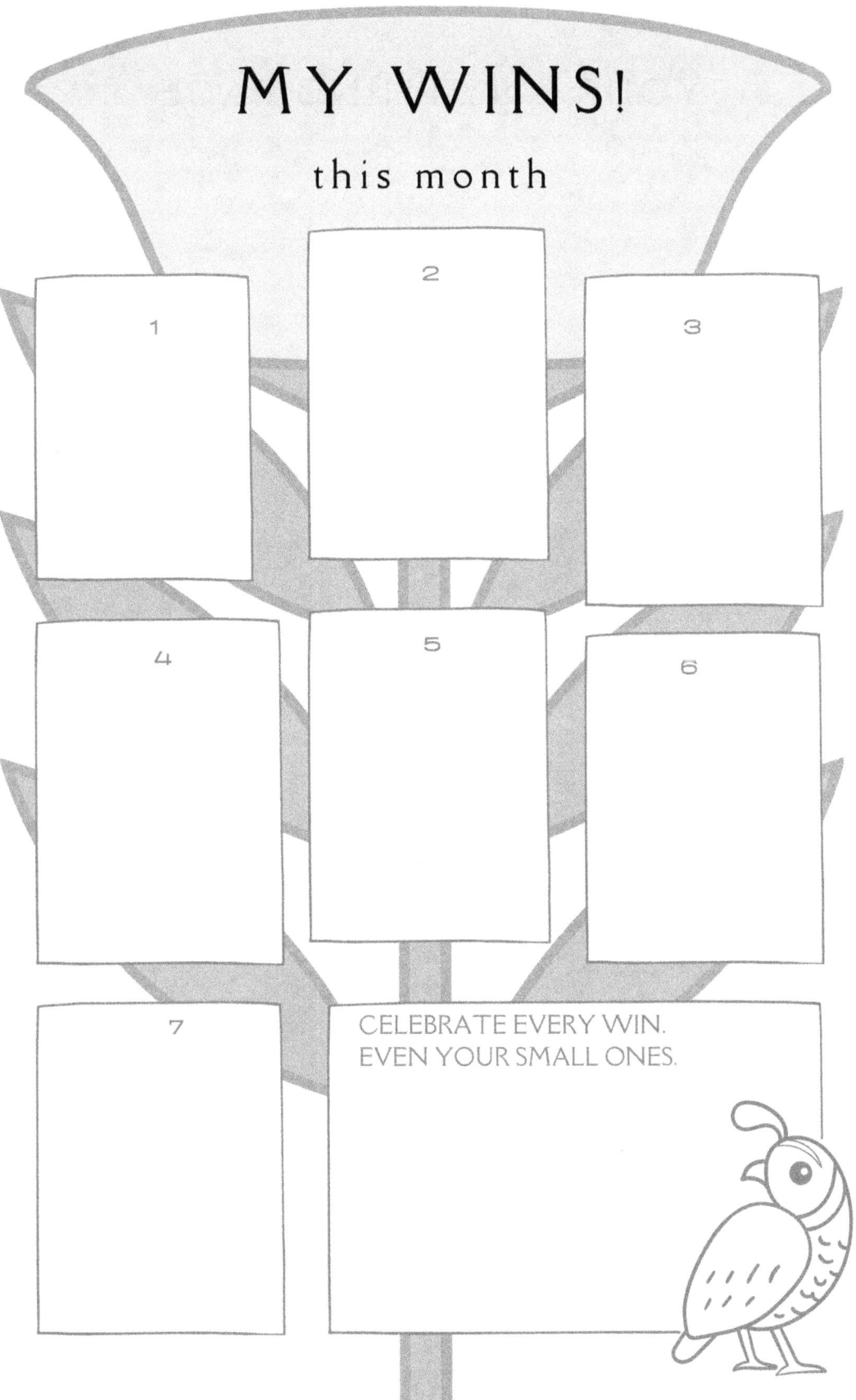

MY WINS!

this month

1

2

3

4

5

6

7

CELEBRATE EVERY WIN.
EVEN YOUR SMALL ONES.

YOUR ANYTHING PAGE

"EVEN IF YOU'RE ON THE RIGHT TRACK, YOU'LL GET RUN OVER IF YOU JUST SIT THERE." —WILL ROGERS

YOUR ANYTHING PAGE

DATE:

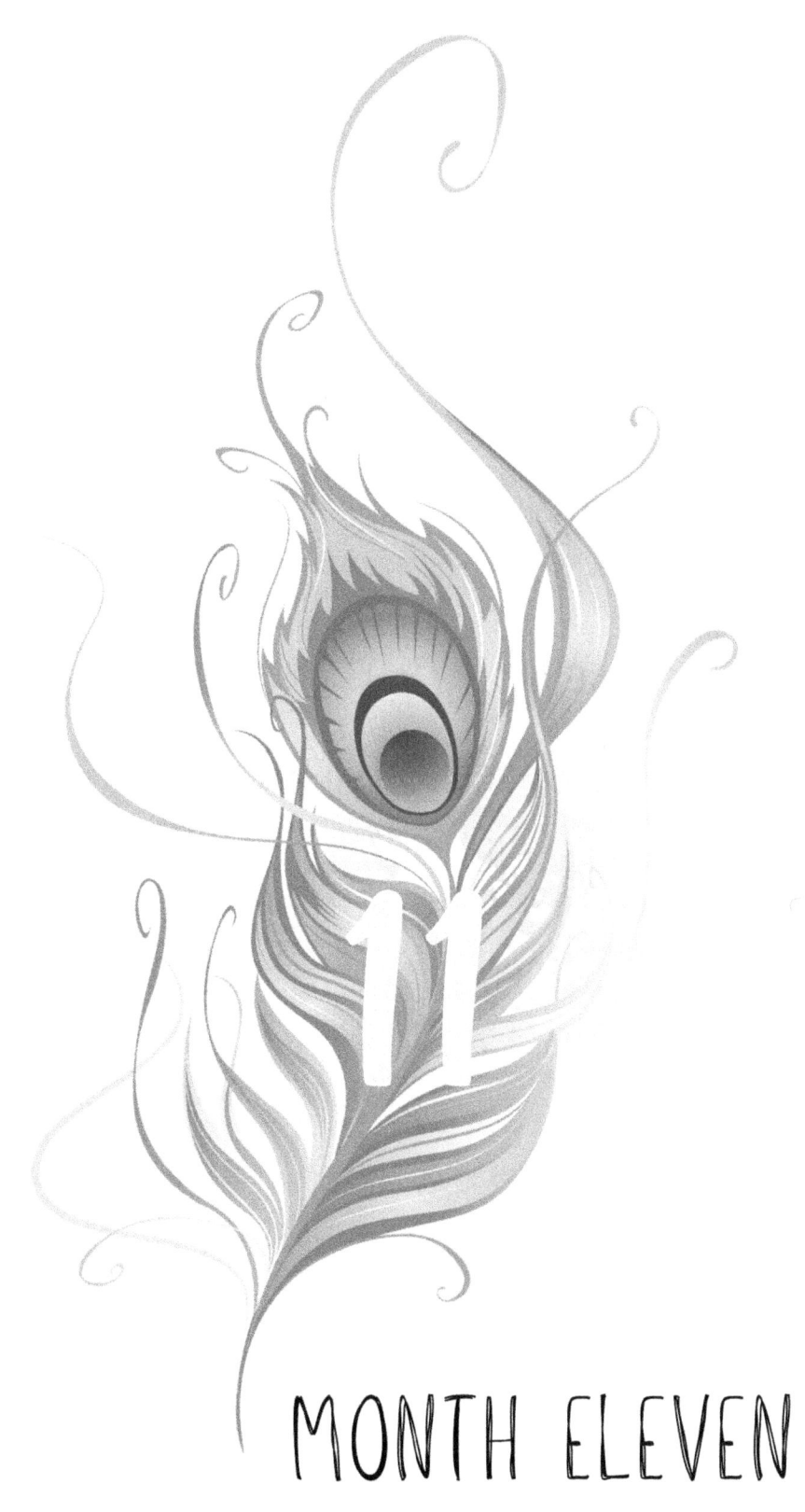

MONTH ELEVEN

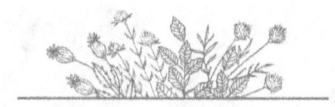

EVERYDAY I AM RENEWED
AND TRANSFORMED. MY LIFE
IS EVOLVING IN FUN AND
EXCITING WAYS.

HABIT TRACKER

MONTH JAN FEB MAR APR MAY JUN JUL AUG SEPT AUG SEP OCT NOV DEC

Track your points to see how you do each month.
Give your self 1 point for every activity square that you fill in.

90 pts ☐   160 pts ☐   My reward for 90≥ _____

120 pts ☐   180 pts ☐   _____

140 pts ☐   My reward for 180≥ _____

_____

_____

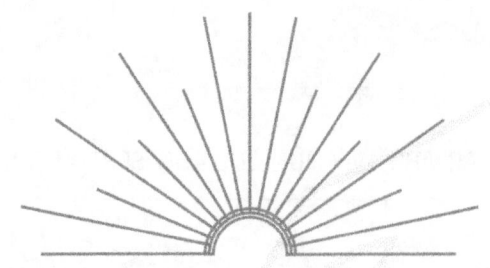

REMEMBER TO CARE FOR YOURSELF

 1    2    3    4    5

 6    7    8    9    10

 11    12    13    14    15

 16    17    18    19    20

 21    22    23    24    25

 26    27    28    29    30

 31   Do something nice for yourself everyday and fill in a heart

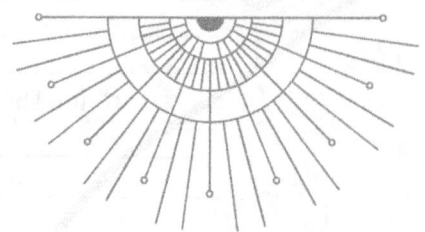

Week 1 - Affirmations / Goals

Date :

Week 2 - Affirmations / Goals

Week 3 - Affirmations / Goals

Date :

Week 4 - Affirmations / Goals

MY WINS!

this month

1

2

3

4

5

6

7

CELEBRATE EVERY WIN.
EVEN YOUR SMALL ONES.

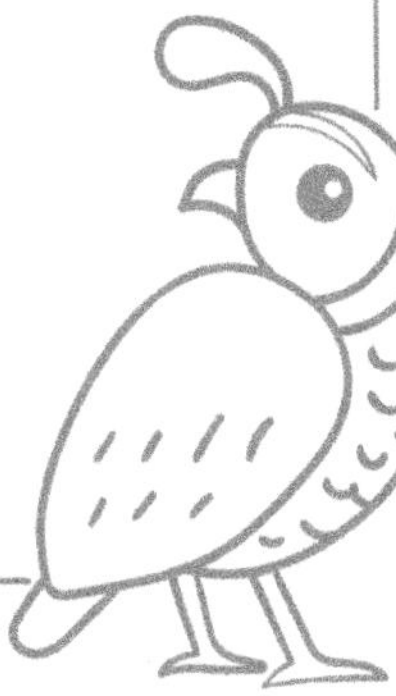

YOUR ANYTHING PAGE

"YOUR LIFE DOES NOT GET BETTER BY CHANCE. IT GETS BETTER BY CHANGE." —JON ROHN

YOUR ANYTHING PAGE

12

MONTH TWELVE

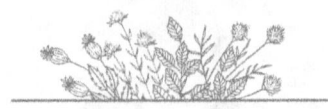

I FOCUS MY ATTENTION
ON FUN AND EVERYTHING
ELSE FALLS INTO PLACE.

HABIT TRACKER

MONTH   JAN FEB MAR APR MAY JUN JUL AUG SEPT AUG SEP OCT NOV DEC

Track your points to see how you do each month.
Give your self 1 point for every activity square that you fill in.

90 pts	☐	160 pts	☐	My reward for 90≥ _____
120 pts	☐	180 pts	☐	_____
140 pts	☐			My reward for 180≥ _____

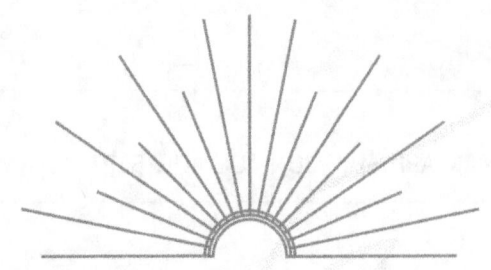

REMEMBER TO CARE FOR YOURSELF

 1  2  3  4  5

 6  7  8  9  10

 11  12  13  14  15

 16  17  18  19  20

 21  22  23  24  25

 26  27  28  29  30

 31

Do something nice for yourself
everyday and fill in a heart

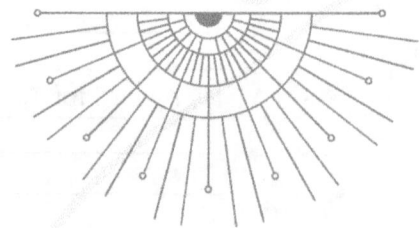

Week 1 - Affirmations / Goals

Date :

Week 2 - Affirmations / Goals

Week 3 - Affirmations / Goals

Week 4 - Affirmations / Goals   Date :

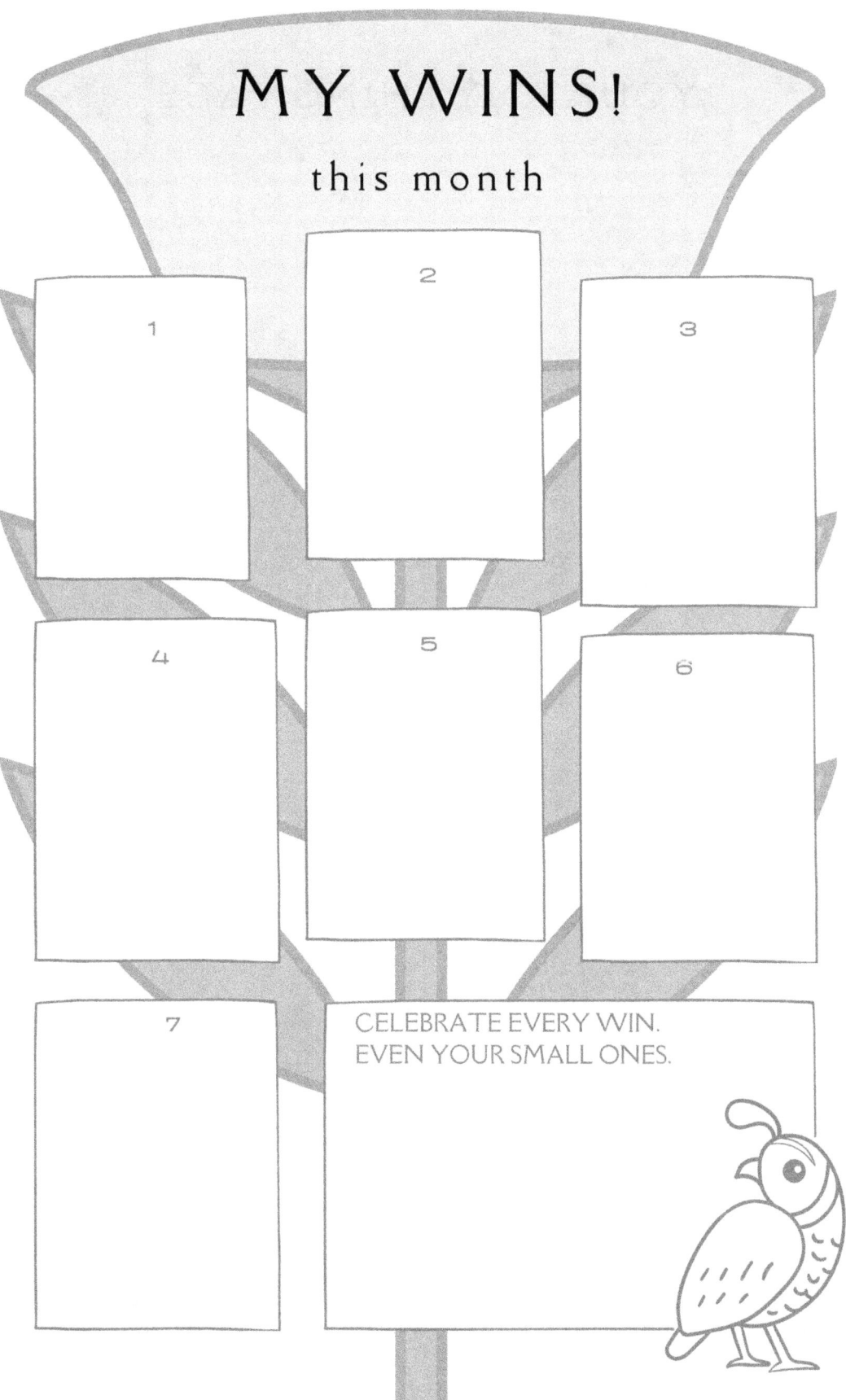

MY WINS!

this month

1

2

3

4

5

6

7

CELEBRATE EVERY WIN.
EVEN YOUR SMALL ONES.

YOUR ANYTHING PAGE

DATE:

YOUR ANYTHING PAGE

DATE:

WHAT'S YOUR STORY?

Do you have an interesting, funny, synchronistic, or other story or event that relates to the topics covered in this book?

Let me know!

Submit your story today for it to be considered for possible inclusion in future editions of this book.

Story guidelines:

Must relate to some process, tool or other from the book.

Must be a true story.

Send inquiries or story submissions here:

Tashai Arts LLC

6516 Monona Dr.

Suite 311

Monona, WI 53716

https://tashai.net

ACKNOWLEDGMENTS

Over the years, many have shared ideas, support or mentoring that has impacted my life, each in their own way. It's impossible to thank everyone and I apologize for anyone I have inadvertently not listed. Please know, that I do greatly appreciate you.

Special appreciation must go to: Joseph Campbell, Dr. Wayne Dyer, Louise Hay, Caroline Myss, Jack Canfield, Patty Aubery, Mike Dooley, Richard Bach, Esther and Jerry Hicks, Abraham Hicks, Darryl Anka and Bashar, James Redfield, Paramahansa Yogananda, Dr John Ryan, Shirley MacLaine, Ram Dass, The 14th Dalai Lama, Edgar Cayce, Kevin Todeschi, Denise Linn, Julia Cameron, James Malinchak, Hal Elrod, Nick Ortner, and Brad Yates.

ABOUT THE AUTHOR

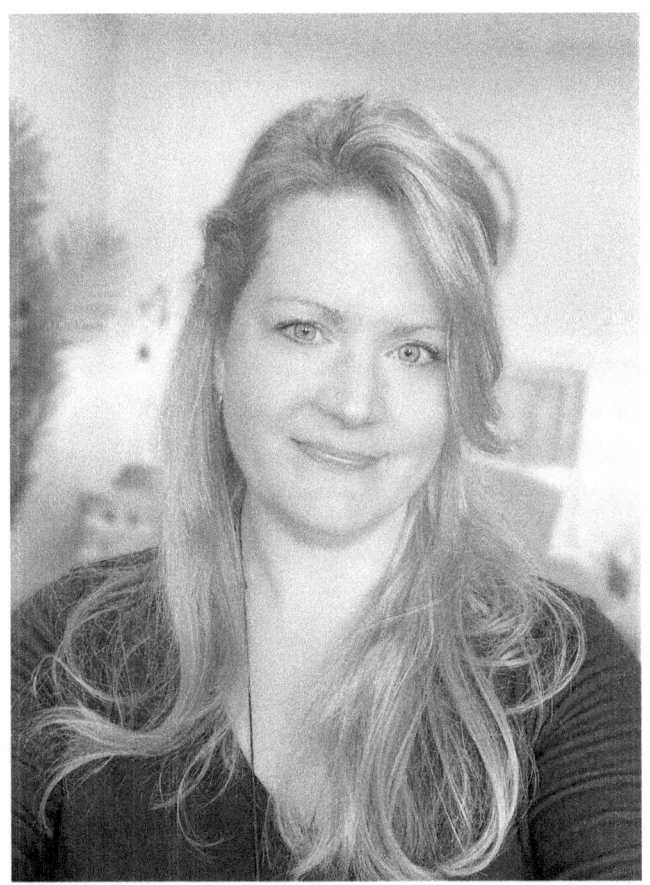

Tashai Lovington is a #1 bestselling author, course-creator, coach, speaker, filmmaker, and spiritual intuitive. She has appeared on public television and her work has been written up in numerous newspapers and periodicals. She was drawn to the study of new consciousness at a very early age which set her on a life-long adventure of discovery. Her work follows in the footsteps of some of the greatest teachers of leading-edge thought. She understands and implements the universal principle of attraction with deliberate intent in all areas of her life. Above all else, she has come to know that our natural state of being is one of joy and that the essence of life is to have fun.

For more of my books, courses, and art, visit my website: https://tashai.net

facebook.com/tashai.lovington
twitter.com/tashailovington
instagram.com/tashai.lovington
tiktok.com/tashai.lov

ADDITIONAL RESOURCES

POPPING THE BUBBLE HOW TO CONNECT WITH YOU INNER GUIDANCE IN 7 DAYS OR LESS

HOME STUDY COURSE

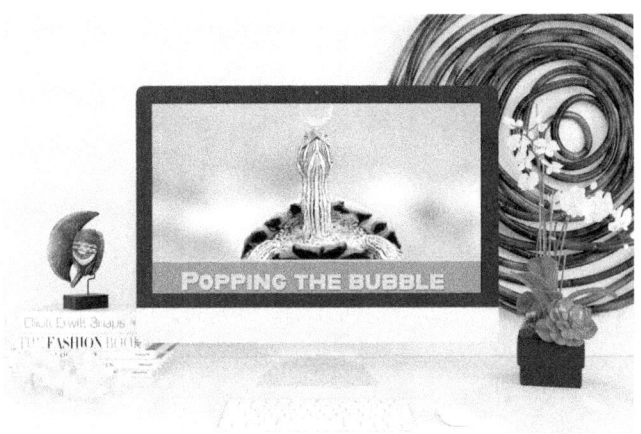

To order go to : https://tashaiarts.samcart.com/products/popping-the-bubble-workshop/

SPECIAL FREE BONUS GIFT FOR YOU

To help you achieve more success, there are FREE BONUS RESOURCES for you at:

https://tashai.net

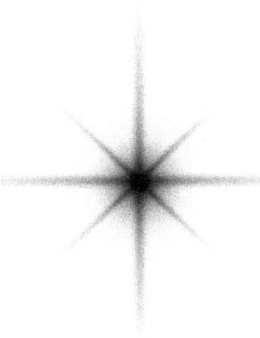